UNDERSTANDING
AUTISM

Professor Katrina Williams is a consultant paediatrician, public health physician and clinician scientist. Katrina has worked and studied in Adelaide, Darwin, Sydney and London and is now the APEX Australia Chair of Developmental Medicine, University of Melbourne; Director, Developmental Medicine, Royal Children's Hospital; and Honorary Research Fellow at Murdoch Childrens Research Institute and is a director of the Australian Advisory Board on Autism Spectrum Disorders. Katrina works as a clinician, service director, educator and researcher specialising in children with neurodevelopmental problems. She has been involved for more than 15 years in initiatives to develop new science, synthesise existing evidence, establish population data and promote evidence into practice and service delivery — especially in relation to autism and other developmental disabilities.

Professor Jacqueline Roberts is the current Director of the Autism Centre of Excellence (ACE) at Griffith University. Jacqui's background in autism stretches back over 30 years. She has worked in Aspect schools for children with autism as a teacher, speech pathologist, principal and senior manager, and has also worked as a consultant and held several appointments at different universities, teaching autism studies and leading research projects. Jacqui is a director of the Australian Advisory Board on Autism Spectrum Disorders, providing input to the board on a national autism research agenda, and served on the DEEWR Students with Disability in Schools Advisory Council from 2010–2013. In 2013 Jacqui received the Asia Pacific Autism Conference (APAC) award for outstanding service to the autism community.

UNDERSTANDING AUTISM

THE ESSENTIAL GUIDE FOR PARENTS

PROFESSOR KATRINA WILLIAMS & PROFESSOR JACQUELINE ROBERTS

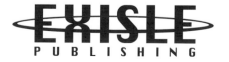

EXISLE
PUBLISHING

Understanding Autism is a very timely book by two of Australia's most respected researchers. Amongst the barrage of information and misinformation about autism, we now have a reference piece aimed squarely at families negotiating the complexity of life, loving and caring for someone who thinks differently and may therefore need a different style of parenting and support in order to reach their potential and to be happy in life. It seeks to answer the fundamental questions about autism as far as our knowledge at this point in time allows us. It does so using the latest evidence and applying it to real-life situations, and this gives parents and carers facts to base their decisions on rather than hearsay or anecdotal stories.

But one of the main reasons I really like this book is that, as the title implies, it is about *understanding* autism, not curing or fixing or forcing change, but recognising that everyone has unique strengths and makes a valued contribution to the fabric of life and community. Families are the first and most important carers in life and play a critical role in making this happen. To do this they need the very best information and the latest research, translated into achievable actions. *Understanding Autism* is a very good place to start this journey.

Judy Brewer
Autism parent and advocate

Although billed as a guide for parents this book would also be of great value to anyone who encounters a child with autism for the first time and needs to begin to understand and best support that child. A decade or so ago, a diagnosis of autism would leave a parent bewildered and isolated — not knowing anything about the disorder and often finding few professionals with sufficient understanding to help. In some rural areas, this might occasionally still be the case but now autism receives much more media attention and, of course, there is the internet. Now the problem is not so much a lack of information as a plethora of information, much of which is, in fact, misinformation. This can be overwhelming for parents (and professionals new to autism) who have no idea whom to trust and where to start in helping their child with autism.

This is the great strength of the book. It is informed by research and is authoritative in tone but is written in an easily accessible style. It uses constructed case studies to illustrate the wide range of characteristics that are found within the autism spectrum, so parents are more likely to see how their child fits into the spectrum. It gives a straightforward account of common interventions in autism, including some that have no scientific backing but are frequently adopted by parents. The book is not judgmental, and recognises that interventions may be adopted for a variety of reasons other than their scientific merit. However, by demystifying much of the technical jargon, and helping parents ask the right questions when evaluating information or approaches, this book helps parents regain control over choosing what is best for them and their child. It also helps remove some of the fear and stress that parents often feel in the beginning, by taking an optimistic (yet realistic) view of the likely development and life chances of children on the autism spectrum.

Professor Rita Jordan BSc. MSc. MA. PhD. C.Psychol. AFBPsS. OBE.
Emeritus Professor in Autism Studies
University of Birmingham, UK

First published 2015

Exisle Publishing Pty Ltd
'Moonrising', Narone Creek Road, Wollombi, NSW 2325, Australia
P.O. Box 60–490, Titirangi, Auckland 0642, New Zealand
www.exislepublishing.com

A CiP record for this book is available from the National Library of Australia.

ISBN 978-1-921966-72-9

Designed by Tracey Gibbs
Typeset in Otari
Printed in China

This book uses paper sourced under ISO 14001 guidelines from well-managed forests and other controlled sources.

10 9 8 7 6 5 4 3 2 1

Disclaimer
This book is a general guide only and should never be a substitute for the skill, knowledge and experience of a qualified medical professional dealing with the facts, circumstances and symptoms of a particular case. The nutritional, medical and health information presented in this book is based on the research, training and professional experience of the authors, and is true and complete to the best of their knowledge. However, this book is intended only as an informative guide; it is not intended to replace or countermand the advice given by the reader's personal physician. Because each person and situation is unique, the authors and the publisher urge the reader to check with a qualified healthcare professional before using any procedure where there is a question as to its appropriateness. The authors, publisher and their distributors are not responsible for any adverse effects or consequences resulting from the use of the information in this book. It is the responsibility of the reader to consult a physician or other qualified healthcare professional regarding their personal care. This book contains references to products that may not be available everywhere. The intent of the information provided is to be helpful; however, there is no guarantee of results associated with the information provided.

CONTENTS

To the parents, children and young
people with autism who have shared
their stories with us.

FOREWORD

Your child or someone else you care for has autism. You might have just found out or you may have known for some time.

In the time we have been working with children, young people and families with autism there has been an explosion of information about autism, including its possible causes and various interventions, and we often hear from families that it is hard to find reliable and relevant information in the one place.

We have written this book to answer the types of questions we are frequently asked. We have created four children and their families and describe their journeys to young adulthood in the hope that this approach brings to life the experiences people with autism have, their many strengths and some of the challenges they face, and also what to expect over time and in different settings.

After addressing some common questions about autism in Chapter 1 and introducing our case studies of children with autism and their families in Chapter 2, the book is then presented chronologically, from the diagnostic assessment through to the types of behaviours and issues faced by a child with autism and their family at each stage of development, with information about the best ways to address these issues. We present resources for further reading at the end of each chapter so relevant information is available as you go. Through these resources and the information we provide about evidence and decision-making in Chapter 10, we also hope to equip you, as parents and carers, with the tools you need to find and assess information for topics we haven't covered, to make best use of new information as it emerges or to form your own opinions about topics we have included.

We hope this book helps you to be the sort of parent or carer you want to be for your child or young person with autism.

A NOTE ON TERMS

The descriptive terms used for autism have changed over the past few decades. For the sake of simplicity, we have used the term 'autism' throughout this book. Other terms you will come across elsewhere include autism spectrum disorder (ASD), autistic disorder or 'classic' autism, autism spectrum condition, high-functioning and low-functioning autism (HFA and LFA), Asperger's disorder, Asperger's syndrome, Asperger's or Aspie. Children with autism may also have been diagnosed with pervasive developmental disorder–not otherwise specified (PDD–NOS) or atypical autism, while some authors refer to 'the autisms'.

Throughout this book we have used the term 'child' in the early sections and then 'young person' in the secondary (high) school section. We realise that in many instances where we have used the word 'child' that the comment also applies to a young person but we have omitted the later clarification to make the book easier to read.

CHAPTER 1

WHAT IS AUTISM?

So, what is autism? Unfortunately, there is no simple answer to this question. Today, autism is seen as a constellation of behaviours indicating problems in social interaction, coping with change, nuances of verbal and non-verbal communication, and restrictive and repetitive behaviours. There are many different behaviours that indicate difficulties in these areas. Individuals with autism, for example, may not initiate interactions with other people, can become very distressed in situations that involve change, or may have highly focused special interests that they pursue to the exclusion of almost all other activities. Despite the enormous amount of research available into the causes of autism and its biological underpinnings, there is no biological test for autism — it remains a behaviourally defined disorder, which means it is diagnosed by watching the behaviours of a child or young person.

It is a truism that no two people with autism are alike. Children with autism can include those with above average intelligence and an intense focus on one area of interest, but with problems in regulating body language and difficulties developing friendships (previously known as Asperger's). At the other end of the spectrum there are children with minimal interest in other people, no ability to communicate and who have self-stimulating behaviours, like watching flickering lights or spinning objects. Some children with autism have very well-developed skills in particular areas, such as creative or number-related abilities, that are sometimes described as savant skills. Having said that, for a child to be diagnosed with autism they need to have social communication problems and restricted and repetitive behaviours of the type and severity described by a diagnostic classification system (more about this later).

Some of the behaviours that are seen in children with autism will respond to intervention more readily than others, varying with the type, severity and reason for the behaviour. For example, a lack of interest in other children may only change slowly, while avoidance of other children because you don't understand them can change quickly as communication or an ability to interpret body language and emotions improves. It is also important to remember that all children with autism will make developmental gains, but the rate and pattern is likely to be different from their peers.

The way we think about autism has changed dramatically over the past few decades. Autism was initially embedded in psychiatry and grouped and named in a similar way to conditions involving thought disorders, like schizophrenia, or disorders of mood and emotion. In the 1970s and 80s, new ways of thinking differentiated autism from psychiatric disorders, and autism began to be thought of as a continuum or 'spectrum' of problems with biological underpinnings.

Two diagnostic classification systems are used internationally to define autism: the *Diagnostic and Statistical Manual of Mental Disorders* (commonly known as the *DSM*) published by the American Psychiatric Association and the International Classification of Diseases (abbreviated to ICD) produced by the World Health Organization. In the early 1990s both the *DSM* and ICD released updated editions that detailed different types of autism, as well as other disorders with some similar but distinguishing features, under the same umbrella term of 'pervasive developmental disorders'.[1,2] During the 2000s, the term 'autism spectrum disorders' became widely used. This term acknowledged the large variation in difficulties and strengths, both in type and severity, which were possible even when the same diagnosis was used. At the same time, autism was being reconceptualised as a neurodevelopmental disorder, with similar underpinnings and assessment approaches needed as with other neurodevelopmental disorders. In 2013, the fifth version of the *DSM* used the term 'autism spectrum disorder' as the official diagnosis for the first time.[3] See also the section about causes below and Chapter 3 about assessment and diagnosis for more detail.

These changes in thinking have had wide-ranging implications for who is diagnosed, the methods used for assessment, the way causes are investigated, the types of interventions that are offered and the location and staffing of services. Changing the way we think about autism from a psychiatric to a developmental framework has brought many advantages and advances. The behaviour of mothers is no longer blamed for causing autism, genetic causes are being identified for some children, interventions are being embedded in developmentally appropriate settings, associations between autism and other neurodevelopmental disorders are being better described and managed, and support throughout a person's life is becoming available through disability services.

WHAT CAUSES AUTISM?

We don't yet have any definite answers but there is emerging consensus that autism is a complex neurodevelopmental problem underpinned by differences in brain connections that are influenced by genes and factors during pregnancy. Many researchers and clinicians believe that the processes leading to the types of problems that are seen in individuals with autism are similar to the processes leading to other neurodevelopmental disorders. The problems seen in autism are increasingly being linked to certain sections of the brain and its interconnections, but not all children with autism appear to have the same sections and interconnections affected, which fits with the differences we see in strengths and problems between children. It follows that the cause may also vary depending on the severity and types of problems that each child has. This is the same for other conditions with an overarching term, like cerebral palsy, which describes many types of motor difficulties of varying severity.

Why do we think that genetics is an important cause of autism? Twin studies in autism have consistently found that identical twins are more likely to have autism than non-identical twins or siblings, which points to genes as a major cause. There are also some genetic differences that have been identified in a minority, albeit an increasing minority, of children with autism. In some instances, a seizure disorder or brain malformation known to be caused by genetic differences has been found. In others, a well-described genetic disorder, like tuberous sclerosis, is known to be associated with higher rates of autism. Recently, scientists have found in individuals with autism more than one of a number of genes that are common to many of us, suggesting that it might be the coming together of common variants that underpins autism (see Table 1 for more information).

Each day we learn more about how DNA and our genes direct how we are made and influence all of our functions by changing the way cells work. Much is also known about the different ways that genes can cause problems, including autism. However, the brain is our most complex organ system so it is not surprising that much is still to be discovered and neurobiology is in its infancy compared to our understanding of other organs and body systems. It will be some time before discoveries made today will change the way we diagnose and manage autism in the future.

Table 1: A brief explanation of the different types of genetic changes that could underpin autism

Common variant genes	These are genes that occur in lots of people but when a number of them come together in the one person they can cause autism. Recent studies have found that about half of all people with autism have common inherited genetic variations. Why would this make sense as a likely cause of autism? It would explain how autistic-like behaviours could occur in individuals who do not have autism. It would explain the amount of variation amongst children diagnosed with autism because there could be different gene combinations that lead to social communication problems and restricted and repetitive patterns of behaviour of different types and severity.
One specific gene that is different (also known as a genetic mutation)	An increasing minority of children with autism are found to have this. There is a deletion or duplication of some part of a gene that turns the gene's message into something different. The deletion or duplication is either inherited or develops spontaneously during the rough and tumble process of fertilisation. The gene can be different in all cells or only in brain cells. If it is only in brain cells, it is harder to detect.
Known genetic disorder with a high risk of autism	A genetic problem is known and a higher proportion of children with that genetic problem have autism. An example is tuberous sclerosis, in which benign tumours grow in the brain and other parts of the body.
Epigenetic changes	The areas between genes previously thought of as non-functioning DNA can change the way genes work even though the gene itself is not different to the gene in other people. The DNA in epigenetic regions can turn genes on and off, either permanently or for short periods.

Understanding that genes are likely to be a big part of the cause of autism doesn't mean that the details are known of how genes or different brain connections cause changes that lead to autism. Many theories exist that would fit in with this understanding, however the specific types of genetic and brain differences and their roles on the causal pathway to autism are still to be discovered.

Work is also underway to find any factors, especially during pregnancy, that increase the risk of autism or protect against it. A lot of change and growth occurs during pregnancy. If at any time blood, carrying oxygen and nutrients, is not delivered to the cells containing DNA, or if unexpected physical factors (such as pressure effects from a twin) damage cells, then differences in development can occur and these could create important differences in the neural pathways during brain development. Hormones, infections and toxins can also influence cellular growth, development and function. We know hormones can change how organs form and function; for example, hormones change the formation of male or female genitalia. We also know that some viruses, like congenital rubella, can damage the brain during early development. However, our understanding of the role of hormones and viruses in creating brain changes that could result in autism is at an early stage. It's also noteworthy that most of these possible pregnancy exposures that could change the way cells work are outside of our control.

Could one factor act in combination with others to cause autism? It is known that some individuals respond differently to various biological challenges, like a change in blood supply or an infection, because of an underlying difference in their DNA. Regions around genes, known as epigenetic regions, have been identified that can change how genes work without altering the actual structure of the gene (see Table 1) and scientists are currently exploring the ways in which epigenetic regions can be changed. It is still early days, though, in terms of knowing how epigenetic regions play a role in causing or preventing health problems in general and autism in particular. Also, for a long time we have known that there is a feedback loop in which our experiences can change our behaviour. It is also possible that this happens in a way that is influenced by our underlying genetics and brain biology. For example, a child who is 'pre-wired' to be less interested in people may avoid interactions, which in turn may switch off some neural pathways, reinforcing this behaviour. This is described as neuroplasticity, where the brain can be influenced by positive or negative exposures. This could explain the improvements brought about by some interventions and brings hope for positive change (see 'Early interventions' in Chapter 5). None of this makes working out the pathways to autism or its causes easy.

An enormous body of work has been published about other possible causes of autism, ranging from dietary factors to immunisation to maternal age. The breadth of these studies reflects the difficulties facing scientists in coming to grips with the factors behind such a complex problem. Many of these theoretical causes are unrelated to each other, while others have no known basis in human biology. Some of the many factors said to be associated with autism, or which are described as theoretical causes, have been disproved, such as the now discredited theory that blamed the vaccine to prevent measles, mumps and rubella (MMR). Others, including specific parts of a child's diet, bowel problems, heavy metals like mercury and lead, air pollution, vitamin deficiencies and the use of common medicines like paracetamol and antibiotics, have not been proven to be causal, despite intensive exploration. For more information about the types of studies that are needed to prove causation and questions to ask to assess suggested causes, see Chapter 10. At present, it appears unlikely that a single external factor will be found to cause autism.

Not all children with autism diagnosed today have identifiable genetic differences. Also, for many of these known differences, not all children with that difference will have autism. This means that we don't yet have the whole story about which genes cause autism and how, but we do know that genes are going to be a big part of the story. Our understanding of other neurodevelopmental disorders that involve more obvious structural brain changes or more easily measured changes in function is rapidly advancing and our understanding of autism is benefiting from this. Discoveries from other areas of science and new technology-driven ways of investigating the brain should mean that progress will be faster in the next five years. Along the way we need to make sure that the multiple theories about the causes of autism are not causing harm and that we think carefully about where finding the causes of autism may lead.

IS AUTISM INCREASING?

This must be one of the most commonly asked questions about autism. There is no doubt that the number of individuals diagnosed with autism has increased over the past five decades. What is less clear, however, is if there are actually more people with the problems of the type seen in autism.

Until the early 1990s, autism was thought to be rare with a prevalence of approximately four in every 10,000. Prevalence is the proportion of a population with a particular condition. From the late 2000s, prevalence as high as more than one in 100, 25 times more common, has been reported.[4] This has raised concerns that there may be an 'autism epidemic' and helped spark the deluge of theories about the likely cause. Equally, it has raised questions about whether the increase in prevalence could be due to factors like changes in diagnostic criteria, increased awareness and the way studies have been conducted.

The way a study is designed and the maths that is used to calculate the final result can have a big impact on reported prevalence. Basing a study in an area that has well-accessed services for autism can lead to finding higher numbers of children, while population-based screening or seeking individuals through service providers, such as hospitals, can affect the outcome of a study. The age of diagnosis can also affect reported prevalence, especially if the age of diagnosis becomes younger and prevalence is reported for preschool children rather than the whole population. Another major factor relating to prevalence is diagnosis. As described above, a diagnosis of autism is generally based on specific criteria set in the classification systems of the day. But the diagnostic classification for autism has changed many times in the last five decades. One major change came with the publication of the fourth edition of the *DSM* in 1994 (*DSM-IV*)[5], in which the diagnosis of autism was broadened, leading to a large increase in reported prevalence soon after.[5] The latest edition, *DSM-5*, published in 2013, has brought further changes that will be discussed in Chapter 3.[6]

There has also been an increase in the awareness of autism in the last three decades. How that influences individuals and families to seek help and the provision of services and diagnostic practises is hard to quantify. All of these things can lead to substantial changes in the number of diagnosed cases even if there has been no real increase in the type of characteristics seen in autism. That is why many experts, from the early 2000s to today, have argued that there may not be a true increase in people with problems of the type seen in autism.

IS THERE A CURE?

Along with the many possible causes of autism have come many potential interventions, some claiming to cure autism or to 'recover' children from autism. There are many learning-based interventions that have been proven to enhance learning, improve communication and modify behaviours (more on this in Chapter 5). There are also many interventions that are known to be effective for problems such as anxiety or poor attention and concentration that are seen in autism but are not autism-specific. With minor modifications, these interventions can have positive effects in children with autism (more on this in chapters 6, 8 and 9). But claims of cures are limited to testimonials and case studies, neither of which are sufficient to say that an intervention is either effective or safe for all children with autism. Claims of 'recovery' are also made in testimonials and have appeared in early intervention studies. Alongside these claims, follow-up studies have found that over time some children no longer meet a diagnosis of autism, while for others their autism-related problems become more severe. It is important to remember that we still don't know all we need to about the natural course of development in children with autism and there is tremendous variability, so it is hard to say whether time or specific interventions are bringing about important changes. We do know enough to say that interventions based on learning are most effective to support development and functioning. However, at present, there is no cure for autism.

WHAT'S AHEAD?

Scientists and clinicians are now trying to make sense of the many different dimensions of autism and using these to try to better understand the genetic mechanisms and neural pathways that result in the common behaviours seen in autism. In doing this they hope to work out why some behaviours occur with other behaviours in some children with autism, but not in others. For example, some children are extremely resistant to change and have very narrow and detailed interests, while others who are resistant to change do not have narrow interests.

In the meantime, accurately identifying children with autism, identifying the types of problems they have, and having that information available for service providers and policy makers is necessary so that adequate services can be made available. The importance of high-quality evidence about prevalence, possible causes, how to accurately diagnose autism, the likely outcomes and whether interventions are effective can't be overemphasised. Nor can the need for individuals and society to embrace difference and provide additional supports when they are needed. If we achieve those things, the future will be better for children with autism and their families.

RESOURCES

International Classification of Diseases criteria for autism
(World Health Organization)

> www.pervasivedevelopmentaldisorders.com/icd-10.htm

> *Diagnostic and Statistical Manual for Mental Disorders*, fifth edition (*DSM-5*) criteria for autism (American Psychiatirc Association)

> www.cdc.gov/ncbddd/autism/hcp-dsm.html

> www.autismspeaks.org/what-autism/diagnosis/dsm-5-diagnostic-criteria

Why vaccines do not cause autism

> www.cdc.gov/vaccinesafety/concerns/autism/

Genetic research and findings

> www.autismspeaks.org/science/initiatives/autism-genome-project

> https://gene.sfari.org/autdb/GS_Home.do

Discussion and figures about autism prevalence

> http://sfari.org/news-and-opinion/viewpoint/2012/population-based-studies-key-for-assessing-autism-prevalence

> www.nimh.nih.gov/about/director/2012/autism-prevalence-more-affected-or-more-detected.shtml

> www.cdc.gov/ncbddd/autism/data.html

> www.autism.org.uk/about-autism/myths-facts-and-statistics/statistics-how-many-people-have-autism-spectrum-disorders.aspx

> www.abs.gov.au/AUSSTATS/abs@.nsf/Latestproducts/4428.0Main%20Features32012

> www.asatonline.org/is-autism-on-the-rise/

Is there a cure for autism?

> www.autism.org.uk/About-autism/Autism-and-Asperger-syndrome-an-introduction/What-are the causes is-there-a-cure/Is-there-a-cure.aspx

> http://raisingchildren.net.au/therapies_services/and_therapies_services.html

> www.fda.gov/ForConsumers/ConsumerUpdates/ucm394757.htm

> www.autism-society.org/living-with-autism/treatment-options/

CHAPTER 2

MEET SOME INDIVIDUALS WITH AUTISM

In this chapter we will introduce some children with autism, and their families, and describe their journey toward becoming young people. These characters have been created from the many different children and families we have met in our work. We hope their stories will illustrate the different types of abilities and strengths that children, young people and families possess, as well as the challenges they can face.

No two children with autism and no two families living with autism will have the same journey through the early years, diagnosis and the school years. It won't only be the type of autism that your child has that influences this experience, it will also depend on where you live, the events of your life and your access to resources (such as family support, community support and intervention services). We hope that reading about these children as they grow up, and their families, will show you that at least some of your experiences are shared by others and provide you with useful information about both common and more specific issues. Like all children, children with autism grow and develop. Your child will make progress in their own way and you will also learn what works and what doesn't for you and your family as time goes on. As we travel from the toddler to the secondary or high school years we'll refer back to these children and their families to highlight some of the different pathways that may be travelled towards important goals and the different types of approaches that can be taken.

Jane

Jane and her family live in a country area just outside a regional centre. Jane is the middle child of three and has an older sister, Jade, and a younger brother, Hayden. Jane's parents separated when her little brother was just a few months old and Jane was four. Jane lives with her mother, Louise, and her brother and sister. Her dad, Mitch, has a new partner and two more children so Jane has a younger half-brother and half-sister. Mitch works as a farm labourer and only makes occasional maintenance payments to Jane's mother, Louise. He has always found Jane's behaviour difficult to manage and his new partner is fearful Jane will hurt her half-siblings so Jane never visits the family and sees her father rarely. This has become more of an issue as Jane has grown older. Jade and Hayden, Jane's brother and sister, spend a lot of time at their friends' houses when they're not at school and avoid inviting their friends to come over because they find Jane too embarrassing.

Since she split up with Mitch, Louise has had a series of boyfriends but no lasting relationship. Some years she has had some seasonal work as a cook and fruit picking but found it difficult to organise care for her children while she was at work, especially for Jane. As a result, she has been unable to work outside the home for several years.

There was nothing unusual about Louise's pregnancy with Jane or with Jane's birth. As a baby Jane was difficult to settle and feed. When Louise started her on solids she would only tolerate very smooth purées and screamed and gagged if there were any lumps. The family GP was not helpful. He couldn't find any physical reason for Jane's sleeping and eating difficulties and made Louise feel she was the cause of the problems.

When Jane was a toddler she preferred bland, pale food and was very reluctant to try any food that was new or different. She loved anything electronic and worked out how to use the television, DVD player and computer. One day Louise found that she had reprogrammed the oven by dragging over a chair to stand on, so she could reach the controls.

Jane, in contrast to both of her siblings, continued to have problems sleeping, which added to family stress. Louise also found toilet-training Jane a challenge, especially when Jane went through a stage of smearing poo.

When Jane was four her mother enrolled her in the small local preschool her older sister Jade had attended, a 30-minute drive away. Jane would start to struggle and protest as soon as her mother packed her bag in the mornings and took her to the car. She liked car travel and looking at the book of road maps and would calm down provided Louise took the usual route until they were close to the preschool when she would start to struggle and protest again. She often had to be forcibly removed from the car and dragged into the preschool. This was very upsetting for everyone.

The preschool staff were concerned about Jane, especially her constant activity and difficulty attending to anything for more than a few minutes. The preschool director suggested Jane should be assessed by the paediatrician who came to the local regional hospital twice a year and saw children in a clinic with the local speech therapist (also called speech and language therapists or speech pathologists).

After a six-month wait for an appointment, Louise took Jane for an assessment. Jane was very anxious and was clingy and tearful throughout. Because attempts to settle Jane were not successful, Louise was asked to fill in some questionnaires and the speech therapist asked Louise to video Jane at home interacting with the family. When the recordings arrived back at the hospital clinic, the speech therapist was able to determine that while Jane's speech was similar to that of other children Jane's age, there were some unusual features. For example, she had particular difficulty joining in conversations, didn't seem to know when and how she should respond, or how to get attention in the usual way.

Jane was diagnosed with autistic disorder. Information gathered highlighted her communication difficulties, and, in particular, the fact that her language and communication skills were much more delayed and disordered than her other skills. Also noted was her lack of interest in social interaction, avoidance of eye contact and her resistance to change and insistence on sameness.

When Jane was six years of age she went to the local primary (junior) school with her brother and sister. Once she settled into school, Jane completed an intelligence (IQ) test with the school guidance officer. This confirmed that her verbal skills were below average for her age while many of her other skills were advanced. For example, when information was presented visually, her problem-solving skills were very advanced for her age, and she could do difficult puzzles easily.

She was in small classes in each year and was lucky to have teachers experienced in special needs most years. Because of Jane's difficult behaviours, the school applied for a teacher's aide (a learning support assistant) to work with Jane in the classroom for a few hours a week as some extra support for her.

Staff at her primary school understood the importance of routine and structure for Jane and set-up daily schedules showing the timetable with pictures. Jane had acquired some literacy skills by the end of primary school and she was able to sight-read but struggled to understand the meaning of what she read so staff again used pictures to illustrate the text to assist her understanding.

When Jane finished primary school Louise enrolled her in the closest local secondary (high) school, some 40 kilometres (25 miles) from the family home. Louise hoped Jane would be able to catch the school bus each day with her older sister, Jade.

The new school was aware of Jane's diagnosis, however there was no transition program to help her settle into secondary school. Jane did not have an individual learning plan and the only information passed on from the primary school was a copy of the most recent application for integration support. Jane's first weeks at the secondary school were a disaster because the uncertainty of the new school environment made her highly anxious. This led to Jane having 'meltdowns' and she would become aggressive towards her peers. Louise decided to keep Jane at home doing distance education for the rest of her first year. A new principal started at the school over the end of year break and he contacted Louise to discuss what the school could do to enable Jane to come back. Jane, Louise and Jane's brother Hayden and sister Jade all worked with the school to develop a program that catered for Jane's strengths and difficulties and planned to gradually reintroduce school as part of her routine from the beginning of the year.

Occasionally things became too much for Jane and she had an outburst, so strategies to manage these occasions were included in her program. Much to the delight of Louise and Jane's teachers, Jane managed the transition to school and was able to successfully complete the year at the secondary school.

When Jane was twelve she started to grow rapidly and at thirteen she was well into puberty and adolescence. Jane had one friend at the secondary school who used to come over sometimes but mostly they were in contact online playing computer games. They spent a great deal of time together and looked out for each other at school. The girls didn't mix with the other students in their class much and while they talked about boys a lot they were not interested in the boys at school.

Jane continued to be very particular about eating and in adolescence she insisted that the food on her plate was separated with no touching allowed. When Jane was in her final year at school, she started a transition program for a technology course at a tertiary college, which she started the following year with some support.

Todd

Todd is an only child. His mother, Jessica, works as a researcher in a university. She was diagnosed with Asperger's disorder shortly after Todd was diagnosed with pervasive developmental disorder–not otherwise specified (PDD–NOS). She recognised many of his characteristics in herself as she was growing up.

Todd lives with his parents in an affluent suburb in a large city. English is spoken at home. Todd's dad, Joseph, works long hours in the city and frequently travels interstate and overseas, so Todd spends much of his time alone with his mother when he's not at school. There is a family history of language and learning problems.

Jessica's pregnancy with Todd went well although she suffered from anxiety for several months. Todd's birth was complicated by a long labour and caesarean delivery, which made the first few weeks more difficult. Jessica reported that Todd walked and spoke early, saying his first words at nine months.

Todd was using one- to two-word phrases at eighteen months but between eighteen and 24 months he stopped using these words and phrases and became distressed with people other than his parents. This made it difficult for Jessica to leave him with anyone aside from his father, who wasn't at home very often when Todd was awake. Todd's hearing was thoroughly assessed and was found to be normal, although until he was three he would block his ears and become distressed on hearing loud sounds, especially if they were sudden or unexpected.

Todd was diagnosed with an expressive/receptive language delay at three, using a speech and language assessment tool. Todd also had a developmental assessment which showed him to have some abilities well above average for his age.

Todd began to speak again when he was three-and-a-half and his language gradually developed. At five years of age he was speaking using two- to three-word phrases. However, he clearly struggled with social understanding and the social aspects of language. He spoke in a soft monotonous voice and rarely initiated conversations with other people unless about his favourite topic, vintage cars. Todd spent many hours arranging his cars in lines according to their size and shape.

The one and only time Jessica held a birthday party for Todd was when he turned four and well before it was due to end he ran and shut himself in his room, refusing to come out until everyone had left.

From the time he was four, Todd attended preschool for a half day, three times a week, with support. He had a learning support aide with him for the first part of each morning. Todd rarely spoke at preschool, but sometimes echoed what was said to him. However, his parents reported that he talked more at home. Todd avoided any interaction with the other children at preschool, playing on his own. Todd had speech therapy once a week for three years and his speech therapist consulted the preschool staff about a communication program for him. Todd also had auditory integration training (AIT) when he was four and was on a gluten- and casein-free diet from the age of four until he started school.

Todd has a great interest in numbers and showed evidence of prodigious calculation skills from a very early age as well as detailed visual recall. After a walk he insisted on drawing all the houses they had passed in order, focusing on the house numbers and drawing in detail the part of the property with numbers on it. He was also able to do mental arithmetic without having ever been formally taught. Before he started school, he could mentally multiply and divide four figure numbers as fast as his parents could work out the answer using a calculator.

As he got older Jessica and Joseph were concerned about some of Todd's behaviours and they requested he also be assessed for autism. The paediatrician noted Todd had some characteristics of autism but not enough for a diagnosis of autistic disorder and his language delay excluded him from Asperger's disorder so when he was four years old Todd was diagnosed with atypical autism or PDD–NOS. Todd was seen by a neuropsychologist who identified that he had a poor auditory working memory, meaning that his ability to retain a list of words or directions he had just heard was less than expected for his age in contrast to his excellent long-term memory and visual memory. The neuropsychologist also found that Todd had no understanding that other people had thoughts and feelings different from his own.

From the time of his diagnosis Todd's family was very concerned about transition to school. Jessica worried that he was not going to cope with school. He had difficulties with change and when stressed or anxious would repeatedly question others but appeared neither to hear nor be satisfied with their answers. The family enrolled Todd at a church-run private school where they hoped he would receive more individual attention and be in a supportive environment.

After his initial difficulties Todd made progress at school and started to participate in small structured group activities in class with certain other children. He learnt school routines and rules and tended to direct or correct other children who failed to comply with these. On some days his repetitive behaviours and rituals were more obvious and interfered with his participation at school. Todd continued to display prodigious calculation skills.

His teacher was concerned about his apparent difficulty with understanding the social behaviour of his classmates and felt this underpinned his lack of interest and ability to interact with the other children. Jessica explained that she had given up asking other children around to play with Todd and that Todd always preferred the company of adults and older children and got on well with one of his older cousins who also had a large collection of vintage model cars.

Throughout his final year at primary school Jessica was very worried about Todd starting secondary school. She and Joseph decided to send Todd to a secondary school run by the same church as his primary school, despite the fact that it was not as close to home and meant Jessica would have to continue to drive Todd to and from school each day.

Fortunately for Todd and his family, the principal at his secondary school had some experience with autism. Some of the teaching staff and the deputy principal had attended a training program designed to enable the school to develop individual programs for students with autism and other needs. The school also had access to a specialised teacher who worked across several schools as an advisor about necessary educational and environmental adaptations. However, not all the teachers in the school were supportive of the program for the students with autism and some refused to make any concessions in their teaching.

While the school provided a range of supports in the classroom and grounds, there were some students who bullied Todd. To address this the school developed a whole-school anti-bullying policy with a range of strategies to combat bullying. Staff were also asked to supervise Todd at all times. After six months the bullying stopped.

Todd had some years at secondary school that were better than others. Much depended on the teachers he had in different subject areas. Todd completed his schooling with high enough marks in his final exams to gain a place at university to study chemical engineering. Although Jessica and Joseph were delighted Todd had managed to get into the university course he wanted, they were worried when they found out that there was no specific support for students with autism. The services that were available were general support services for students with disabilities but Todd did not feel this was relevant for him and refused to register for special support, but he did find a staff member in the maths department who offered individual supervision.

Siew

Siew's parents, Kenneth and Hong Yuan, met at university in Australia, where they were both enrolled as international students. Hong Yuan studied economics and Kenneth computer science. Kenneth was from Singapore and Hong Yuan was from Taiyuan in northern China. They returned to China after completing university and married and then lived for some years in Singapore with Kenneth's family.

Siew was a very placid baby. He slept well, fed well and was usually happy or content. The family was delighted to have a first-born boy and there were celebrations in Singapore and China.

When Siew was two years old and Hong Yuan was pregnant with their second child, the family decided to move to Australia permanently. However, after the family moved to Australia, they became concerned about Siew. He was no longer saying some words he had in Mandarin at eighteen months of age and he had become quite withdrawn and distant. Leila was born three months after the family arrived in Australia.

Six months after the move Zhen Zhu, Hong Yuan's mother and Siew's grandmother, came to stay with the family to help with Siew and his little sister Leila. Hong Yuan hoped to return to work when Leila was twelve months old and depended on her mother for child care. Kenneth worked full time and long hours for a big multinational company. It was a busy time for the family with a new baby and adjusting to their new life.

It was only after Leila was born and Zhen Zhu arrived that Hong Yuan and Kenneth really started to worry more about Siew's development, especially when they noticed the difference between their two children. Also, Hong Yuan compared Siew to the children of her friends and began to realise there was something very different about him.

Zhen Zhu, however, believed that Siew's lack of speech was quite normal and she refused to accept that there were problems with his development, which made it difficult for Kenneth and Hong Yuan to discuss their concerns with her. Zhen Zhu said that one of her brothers didn't talk until he was five years old and there was nothing wrong with him.

Siew's parents talked to their local doctor about their concerns and he referred them to a paediatrician for assessment when Siew was three years old. The paediatrician completed a standardised developmental assessment and noted that in some areas of development, such as motor skills, Siew was much better than in other areas, like communication and social development. During the assessment Siew became very distressed and covered his ears when a truck started backing up outside making a high-pitched beeping sound. He also ran around the room on tiptoes and flapped his hands when he was excited. Hong Yuan told the paediatrician Siew had a favourite DVD he watched repeatedly.

Based on observing Siew's behaviour, the developmental assessment and talking to Hong Yuan and Kenneth, the paediatrician made a provisional diagnosis of autistic disorder and recommended a repeat visit to assess his progress in six months' time. The paediatrician also suggested Siew have a communication assessment and speech therapy to help improve his communication skills and gave Hong Yuan and Kenneth contact details for the service to call to arrange early intervention and also the contact details and website for the local autism association. The paediatrician told them that it is very difficult to predict how children with autism develop and mentioned that he may need specialist support for many years to come. When Kenneth and Hong Yuan told Zhen Zhu what the paedictrician had said, she flatly refused to accept there was anything wrong with Siew and repeatedly suggested that they return to China for some traditional medicine. Hong Yuan and Kenneth found it difficult to cope with this pressure.

Hong Yuan and Kenneth had decided that once they were in Australia they would speak English at home, however Chinese (Mandarin) was used a lot after Zhen Zhu came to stay with the young couple. When they spoke to Siew's speech therapist about it she recommended that they speak their first language at home (Mandarin) as that would be best for Siew's communication development.

Hong Yuan enrolled Siew in a specialised playgroup for children with autism, which they attended two mornings a week. At this time Siew had very little speech. Staff at his playgroup noted that he babbled occasionally in 'Chinese' but rarely used language functionally. On one occasion at the playgroup he was heard to say 'mum' and on another 'no', but he had not been heard to use English words in any other context. Siew looked at his mother and put his arms up when he wanted her help or to be picked up. He rarely initiated interaction at other times. He didn't look at his peers unless they stood near him and then he liked to touch their hair. When a teacher or parent played with action–response toys and then stopped he did not make eye contact but continued to stare at the toy. Siew communicated by giving objects, reaching, touching and dropping objects and crying. He communicated more at home, usually when he wanted comfort or a favourite toy, than at playgroup.

Siew's speech therapist introduced visual aids to help Siew communicate and worked with both his parents and the playgroup staff so that any strategies used were consistent across all the settings. She had to spend some time convincing Siew's grandmother that visual aids were helpful. Siew was better at communicating using his visual system than speech. Although he developed a growing vocabulary, there were times when he found it easier to express himself non-verbally. Hong Yuan also found a picture schedule very useful to explain to Siew any changes in their usual routine.

When Siew was nearly five, his parents started to look at different primary school placements for him. They found it difficult to decide if he should go to a specialist school for children with autism or a regular school. Hong Yuan talked to other mothers at her parent support group and was very confused because there were so many different opinions. Finally, after visiting several schools near their home and a school for children with autism some distance away (attendance would require an hour in the school taxi each way morning and afternoon), Hong Yuan and Kenneth decided to enrol Siew in the local primary school. They had an interview with the principal and found out that the school would apply for extra resources for a teacher's aide to help Siew, who would work with him for three hours each day.

Siew started primary school initially for three hours each day when the teacher's aide was there. The hours gradually increased to a full day as he settled into school. Hong Yuan was able to continue in full-time work with Zhen Zhu helping to look after both children. Hong Yuan found it difficult to get to the parent support group meetings which were usually held during working hours. The family were able to join in social activities with other families from the group at weekends and Hong Yuan formed friendships with several of the other mothers. Zhen Zhu gradually stopped worrying that contact with other children with autism at these occassions would set Siew back. By the time Siew finished primary school he could read and write in both English and Mandarin. His results were mixed even within subject areas, for example, he was good at calculation in maths but found it difficult to do language-based maths problems. He wasn't really part of a friendship group, although there were a couple of kids in his class who looked out for him.

Siew went to the local secondary school, which was much larger than his primary school, and things became very difficult, despite having an assistant allocated to support him for three hours each day. He found it hard to cope with both the academic side and the social aspects of school. Having his teacher's aide with him much of the time tended to make him stand out more and reduced any chance of him fitting in with the other students. Siew became very anxious at secondary school; he was unable to follow the timetable when his aide wasn't there and was unable to cope even when she was if there were unscheduled changes. He developed self-injurious behaviour and would hit his head with his hands when distressed. A behaviour specialist from the education department was called in. Siew also found it increasingly hard to cope in a noisy crowded environment, like school assembly. Over time his mood and behaviour became more worrying and he started hitting his head with closed fists and making loud noises. The school requested Hong Yuan and Kenneth keep Siew at home while they worked on a program for him to manage his behaviour at school with a view to gradually re-introduce Siew to school.

One of Hong Yuan friends in the parent support group recommended her son's school, where there was a specialist unit for students with autism. Her own son was doing well there. Hong Yuan and Kenneth moved to be able to access the best option for Siew's education. Siew was much more settled in the specialist unit, which made things much easier at home too.

Siew completed secondary school in the specialist unit. A year before he finished school, staff working with Hong Yuan and Kenneth started to prepare for his transition to the local technical college. At the technical college Siew enrolled in a horticultural course which included work experience three mornings a week on a council work crew maintaining local parks and gardens.

John

John lives with his dad Mike, mum Sue and one older brother Sam. Mike works as a mechanic and drives to work each day. Sue wanted to go back to some part-time work once John and Sam were at school but jobs were hard to find in the outer suburbs where the family lives and the family can only afford one car.

Sue's pregnancy with John was uncomplicated although she found it hard coping with Sam, who was a very lively toddler, during the last three months. Sue was terrified when John had his first seizure at ten months of age. She rang Mike who told her to call an ambulance. After the first seizure John had an electroencephalogram (EEG) and Mike and Sue were told he had epilepsy.

When John was two-and-a-half the specialist at the teaching hospital who managed his epilepsy was concerned about John's lack of communication and social development and referred him for a developmental assessment. John was assessed over two days by a multidisciplinary team led by a paediatrician who specialised in developmental disability. The team assessing John included a speech therapist, an occupational therapist, a psychologist and a social worker. All aspects of John's development were assessed using a combination of formal standardised tests, observations of John and a discussion with Mike and Sue. The assessment confirmed Mike and Sue's worst fears — John's development was very delayed compared to other children his age, especially his ability to communicate and relate to other people. The assessment by the occupational therapist at the hospital confirmed that he had some unusual sensory characteristics. He disliked light touch and the sensation of clothing on his skin but liked deep pressure, which seemed to be calming for him. Mike and Sue reported that at home he liked to lie under heavy cushions and enjoyed physical play with his dad, especially being swung around. It was also noted that John became distressed with any change, like sitting in a different chair. Sue and Mike were also concerned about John's tendency to eat things he picked up from the floor or outside which were not food. The paediatrician explained this was something that some children did.

John was diagnosed with autistic disorder and severe intellectual disability. Because John also suffered epilepsy from a young age, neuroimaging using MRI was also performed, but no abnormality was found.

The assessment team at the hospital explained to Mike and Sue that John would need specialist health and education support. They explained the options for management and recommended Mike and Sue start an early intervention program as soon as possible.

In the second half of the year when John was four he attended preschool for three mornings a week with support from his early intervention professional. As he gradually learned skills she worked less with John directly and more with the whole group, always moving John towards participating more independently. He learnt to sit with the other children, on the outside of the group, for 'mat' time for ten minutes at a time and to choose a song for the group to sing with the teacher when offered a choice of two using a picture board. He learnt to give his teacher an 'I want a break' card when the noise was too much for him and was able to go to a special quiet corner the preschool staff had set up for him with lots of big soft cushions and some of his favourite books to flip through, or to jump on a small trampoline also set up for him to use. These activities helped him to calm down and regulate his emotions and stress.

Sue found it very hard to talk to her other friends about what was happening with John and her family, and found it upset her to join in with their planned mother and child activities. She joined a parent support group for parents of children with autism, which she found very helpful.

The mothers in the support group were trying lots of different therapies and interventions and some of them were convinced that their child was allergic to wheat and dairy and this was the cause of their autism. Sue thought it was important to try to remove these foods from John's diet and hoped this would help him.

Sue found it hard to toilet-train John. He seemed to be unaware of the need to go to the toilet and wore nappies for the first four years of his life, but once Mike and Sue noticed him beginning to fidget in a certain way before he urinated or had a poo they spoke to John's early intervention worker, and when they followed the plan she developed he was out of pull-up nappies after eight months.

In the year John turned five his early intervention therapist started talking to Mike and Sue about possible schools for John. It was clear by then that he had great difficulty understanding language and that he relied heavily on visual information to understand his environment. John didn't communicate much with other people. He rarely initiated communication unless he wanted something, however he liked to be close to his parents and his brother. He learnt to use a visual communication system with his family and the preschool staff, consisting of laminated cards and pictures, either drawings or photos of familiar things and activities. He also used and understood a few hand signs such as the sign for 'more' and 'finished'. John only responded sometimes when those around him tried to communicate with him and it was hard to know whether he did not understand or was just not interested.

Mike and Sue wanted John to go to the same local school as his brother, Sam, but the professionals they spoke to thought he would struggle in a regular school. Sue and Mike visited the local regular school and the nearest special school, and decided to enrol John in the special school. He started integrating into school when he turned five and started school full-time six months later. John went to and from school each day in a taxi with four other children who were all collected from home. He spent a long time in the taxi each day, sometimes as much as 45 minutes each way if the traffic was heavy.

At school John was assessed and an individual learning plan was developed. John's teacher, Janet, noted that John was attracted to flashing lights, had very limited receptive and expressive communication and that rolling (and eating) playdough was one particular special interest. He also showed an interest in the telephone directory in the office and a set of books in the classroom he would flip through repeatedly. At school John tended to be withdrawn and self-absorbed and displayed very limited social skills. He also did not usually engage or interact with adults or with his peers for a social purpose and usually found being in the same area or close to his peers quite challenging. If another student came close, he would usually move away. When John started school, Janet incorporated his visual communication system into the system used in the classroom and also used some of his special interests to engage John in learning new skills and to address unwanted behaviours.

Unfortunately, communication between the school and Mike and Sue was not good. Although they were invited to attend a meeting to plan John's education a few months after John started school, they had very little input into John's program and noted that Janet, the teacher, did not seem very interested in how much of John's program was being worked on at home. On one occasion they found out from the driver of John's taxi that one of the other children in John's class had lots of behaviour problems and had been hitting out at the other children and injuring himself. They worried about this and about John being hurt.

John continued on an anticonvulsant medication through primary school. He was now having one to two seizures a year, rather than one each month and his parents were very worried about how the school would manage if John had a fit. They checked with the school and found out that the staff were trained to manage seizures and that strategies were in place, which reassured them John would be safe.

By the time John was twelve he had a communication folder that contained photos and drawings that he used to request an object or activity, however he usually required a verbal prompt 'show me what you want' to do this. He only asked for a limited range of things using his communication system such as 'drink', 'biscuits', 'crackers' and 'sandwich'.

John continued to attend the special school, which provided schooling for children with disabilities from five to eighteen years of age. As he got older, he sometimes injured himself hitting his head with his hands or against furniture and walls when he was stressed and agitated.

The special needs school John attended had a unit in a regular secondary school designed to give students the opportunity to spend time with non-disabled peers, but in reality there was limited meaningful engagement with students in the regular secondary school. John and his class of eight joined the regular students once a week for a whole-school assembly, for sports classes and for some art and home economics activities but there was very little social interaction and no lasting relationships formed.

The secondary school staff started working with Mike and Sue in John's final year of school when he was seventeen to find a suitable program for him to move to when he finished school. Nothing suitable was found before he was eighteen, so he stayed at the school while the staff and Mike and Sue continued their search. Before the end of the year John started a supported employment day program four days a week.

CHAPTER 3

ASSESSMENT AND DIAGNOSIS

Diagnosis is usually a critical time for families and many parents talk about their lives before and after their child was diagnosed with autism. Children and families come to assessment and diagnosis via different pathways. In general, an assessment will have been arranged because you or others have concerns about your child's development or behaviour.

While you may want to know 'Does my child have autism?', health professionals will generally initiate a broad assessment process to gather information about your child's overall strengths and weaknesses. The aim is to understand your child in relation to expected development for their age, their usual environments, and both the cause and effect of any unwanted behaviours. The assessment will also explore if there could be any underlying biological reasons that explain your child's problems with developmental progress and behaviour. All of this information will be used to develop a profile of your child, to decide whether or not they have autism, and to assist with short and longer term planning.

All the four children and their families in this book had different paths toward an assessment.

> John was directed for a developmental assessment by a specialist he was seeing for his epilepsy and was assessed by a multidisciplinary team led by a paediatrician. Siew's parents took their concerns to their GP, who referred him to a paediatrician.

Diagnostic services are not always available locally, especially for families in rural and regional areas, and even in metropolitan areas there may be long waiting lists for assessment.

> Jane's family GP dismissed her mother's concerns and it wasn't until preschool staff raised concerns that Jane was put on the waiting list for a visiting assessment clinic, leading to a delay between concerns first being raised and diagnosis.

A staged process of assessments can clarify identified difficulties, help plan tailored interventions and link to further assessments as needed.

> Todd's diagnosis occurred over time, with an initial diagnosis of a language delay with superior intellect, but further assessment when social problems emerged led to a diagnosis of atypical autism.

Some children with autism won't be diagnosed until they're in primary (junior) or even secondary (high) school when their social difficulties become evident.

HOW IS AUTISM DIAGNOSED?

There is no biological test for autism. Autism is diagnosed by hearing about and watching behaviours and developing an understanding of your child's abilities and how they get along in different situations and settings. The way your child communicates, their interest in others, and unwanted behaviours that are interfering with their and your life are of interest. Whether behaviours coexist with other neurodevelopmental problems, such as a language problem or attention and concentration problems (for more information see Chapter 7), and whether there are any underpinning medical issues, like tuberous sclerosis, is important to assess. Experts will also take into account how the behaviours and other abilities have changed over time, and whether a behaviour or developmental pattern is seen in multiple settings rather than just in one, with behaviours in multiple settings being more likely to be neurodevelopmental. They will also look at the severity of any problems.

While very few diagnostic tests are perfect, diagnosing behaviourally defined disorders is prone to more error than those with well-established biological markers. With every change in behavioural diagnostic classification systems (like *DSM-5* and ICD-10) developers are trying to increase the accuracy of diagnosis, and to best align a diagnosis with identification of an underlying cause, choice of the best interventions and prediction of what the future will bring. To do this, most diagnostic systems have in-built rules that need to be followed before a diagnosis can be given. Some of the rules indicate the type and number of behaviours, also known as criteria, that need to be present. Others identify additional testing that needs to be done to be sure that the behaviours cannot be explained as appropriate for a child's developmental level. Yet others describe what has to be excluded before a diagnosis can be made.

The specific cause of autism is still not known in most children and because of the wide variation in the types of difficulties and strengths and in the degree of severity seen in children with autism, a diagnosis does not by itself give us the information we need to understand what the future holds or to recommend interventions and services. It does direct some of the investigations we do, but it isn't enough to tailor investigations for each child. Most importantly, a diagnosis of autism alone is not enough to enable everyone to understand your child's specific needs and abilities.

A diagnosis can still be helpful because it enables people to talk about and understand the types of difficulties your child is experiencing.

In many countries a diagnosis is required to access services, or funding for services, that you and your child need.

THE DIAGNOSTIC ASSESSMENT

An ideal diagnostic assessment is multifaceted and includes your account of your child's strengths and difficulties, information about your child from others who care for them, observations of your child by professionals, and standardised tests of language and other abilities. Possible medical explanations for any presenting behaviours will also be explored. As such, the gold standard assessment for autism and other developmental concerns is often called a 'multidisciplinary assessment', which means it involves clinicians from different disciplines, like speech pathology, psychology and medicine.

During the assessment you will be asked to describe your child's strengths and difficulties, any concerns you have with their behaviour, including how long you have been aware of the behaviours, and whether they come and go over time or in different settings. You will also be asked if your child has responded to any interventions you may have tried. Accounts from other people who care for your child will also be sought, like their child-care workers. In addition, all your child's strengths and difficulties will be assessed in terms of their trajectory, or change over time, rather than as static or fixed. Information about any gains or deterioration in development or behaviour over time will also be gathered, and compared to gains in other areas.

An assessment can also include the use of diagnostic tools, such as current versions of the Autism Diagnostic Interview™ (ADI), the Autism Diagnostic Observations Schedule™ (or ADOS), the Childhood Autism Rating Scale™ (CARS), the Gilliam Autism Rating Scale (GARS), the Developmental, Dimensional and Diagnostic Interview (3di) or the Diagnostic Interview for Social and Communication Disorders (DISCO) (see Glossary for information about these diagnostic tools). However, the use of diagnostic tools in isolation is not sufficient for a diagnosis to be made, nor are they required in order to make a diagnosis.

Once information has been gathered to clarify your child's strengths and difficulties, the assessment team will think about whether there are any patterns emerging in their developmental pathway and behaviours. These patterns of behaviour and development are then compared with diagnostic criteria and rules as described in the international classification systems *DSM* or ICD.

If further information is needed then investigations will be planned, further assessments decided, and whether a period of intervention would assist in making the diagnosis will also be considered. In autism, information about response to intervention can be very helpful. For example, if a child starts to join in with their peers following speech therapy, it could mean that their difficulties were due to a speech disorder rather than a lack of interest in peers. This may mean that autism is not the most appropriate diagnostic label, depending on whether other criteria are satisfied. Similarly, a behaviour like insistence on watching one program repeatedly would not indicate 'highly restricted, fixated interests that are abnormal in intensity or focus' as required for criteria B3 of the *DSM-5* if the child easily switches attention when other activities are offered.[1]

DIAGNOSTIC CRITERIA AND RULES

Of the two main classification systems used internationally, the *Diagnostic and Statistical Manual of Mental Disorders* released a new edition (*DSM-5*) in 2013. The only diagnosis possible using the *DSM-5* is autism spectrum disorder, whereas the diagnoses of childhood autism, atypical autism, Asperger's syndrome, pervasive developmental disorders, other or unspecified, are still possible using ICD-10.

The behaviours that are required for a diagnosis of autism using *DSM-5* and described in criteria A and B are of two types: 'persistent deficits in social communication and social interaction across multiple contexts' and 'restricted, repetitive patterns of behaviour, interests or activities'.[2] Meanwhile, ICD-10 requires problems with three types of behaviours: 'reciprocal social interaction, communication, and restricted, stereotyped, repetitive behaviour'.[3] For the rest of this discussion we use *DSM-5* to illustrate diagnostic processes because it is commonly used and the most recently revised.

A diagnosis using *DSM-5* must meet certain rules. As well as information about behaviours required for diagnostic criteria, information will be gathered to assess whether the problem has presented at the right age, whether other diagnoses have been excluded, and whether the problems are out of keeping with your child's level of ability, not just for their age. These rules exist in an effort to improve the accuracy of a diagnosis.

For a diagnosis of autism, developmental and behavioural problems must: (1) be present from early in life; (2) 'cause clinically significant impairment in social, occupational or other important areas of current functioning'; and (3) not be better explained by intellectual disability, also known as intellectual developmental disorder.[4]

In addition, whether the diagnosis of autism is 'associated with a known medical or genetic condition or environmental factor' must be specified. This is important because we know that children with environmental risk factors or known genetic or medical conditions may need interventions that are different or additional to those without such factors. When assessing the likelihood of inherited (genetic) or other causes of your child's difficulties, professionals will ask about family history and conception, pregnancy and the birth (see also Chapter 1).

> For Todd there was a family history of mild language delay and disorder and learning difficulties, and Todd also has one cousin with a diagnosis of mild intellectual impairment.

The *DSM-5* has introduced severity levels to be included in the assessment. A severity level should be applied to both the social communication criteria and the restricted, repetitive behaviours criteria. The severity for each of these categories of difficulties can be described as one of three levels: 'requiring very substantial support', 'requiring substantial support' and 'requiring support'. It is hoped that these severity categories will increase the usefulness of the diagnosis but this has not yet been established. How well these categories work in creating meaningful subgroups of individuals with autism, either for research or for service planning, is also not yet known.

KEY ASSESSMENT COMPONENTS

Your child may find it difficult to settle in a different environment and not join in the tasks expected for an assessment, so the first part of any assessment will be trying to make your child at ease and engaged. Sitting your child on your lap and allowing them to play with familiar toys may help your child feel more relaxed at the beginning of an assessment.

> Jane did not respond to any attempts made by the doctor or the speech therapist to engage her in interaction. She avoided looking at them and wrapped herself in her mother's skirt. Louise tried coaxing Jane with some of her favourite treats and eventually she settled on her mother's lap and started to look at some of the test items the clinicians showed her but she did not speak or respond to any directions. She did smile and showed some interest in the bubble wand and tried to catch the bubbles as they floated past.

LANGUAGE AND COMMUNICATION ASSESSMENT

A communication, speech and language assessment is a vital part of the diagnosis. It is necessary to interpret your child's behaviours in terms of their ability to understand and communicate, but it is also important for other reasons. It can be extremely helpful in developing an understanding of the cause of behaviours and, in doing so, provides opportunities for starting effective interventions (see Chapter 5).

Assessing your child's communication will involve learning about their understanding of words and speech (called 'receptive language' or comprehension) and their understanding of non-verbal communication, such as gestures and expressions. The assessment will also involve learning about how your child expresses themselves and the speech and language they use (verbal communication) and other non-language ways they adopt to express themselves, such as noises, gestures, signs or pictures (non-verbal communication). The assessment will also consider why your child communicates (are they asking for things or sharing information?), and what they communicate about (is it only their special interest?).

If your child understands and uses spoken or written words, the assessment will also consider your child's mastery of the rules that govern language in relation to expected ability for age. Aspects of your child's language development may be delayed, that is, at a level that is expected for a younger typical child, and aspects of their language development might be different or unusual for children of any age (also called disordered). Characteristics of language development often seen in autism include uneven language development with better ability to speak than to understand and high levels of repeating what has been said either immediately or after some time has passed. Children, including those with autism, use imitation to varying degrees as they develop language. In typical children the use of imitation gives way to the use of rules to produce 'correct' sentences as they grow and mature. In children with autism this process can be disrupted and they will continue to use imitation after typically developing children have stopped. If imitation occurs in speech after the age of three, it is referred to as 'echolalia'. It is usually associated with problems understanding language and does not only occur in autism, but is common in the speech of children with autism who learn to talk. Children with autism are very likely to have some elements of disordered language and by definition have communication difficulties.

> For Jane, although her speech was similar to that of other children her age, there were some unusual features in content, where she repeated what people said to her. Her language also sounded memorised or rote-learnt. The speech therapist also noted Jane had problems understanding what was said to her, especially when language was more complex (for example, 'If you

put your toys away you can come with me to get the pizza') or abstract ('Well … get a wriggle on, what are you waiting for?'). The speech therapist also noted that the aspect of communication Jane had most difficulty with was the interpersonal use of communication. For example, Jane would ask her brother for something without looking at him or moving close to him.

Ideally, a communication assessment should occur in different settings and include information from you about how your child communicates at home, at child care or school and in the community. When it is not possible for professionals doing the assessment to observe your child in those settings, videos can be helpful.

Louise explained that Jane spoke quite a bit at home and could remember big chunks of dialogue and sound effects from her favourite DVDs. Louise filled in several questionnaires about Jane's communication and the speech therapist asked Louise to video Jane at home interacting with the family. She suggested times like meal times and bath times when Jane was more likely to communicate with her mum and other family members.

This can be a very helpful supplement to an assessment, and can also assist if you feel that your child's performance on the day of the assessment was different than usual, perhaps due to anxiety or other factors.

Various communication assessment tools are used for children of different ages and different aspects of communication assessment.

For young children like John and Siew who are non-verbal, the focus would be on assessing their level of understanding any form of communication, for example noting that they may understand visual information, like a picture of a milkshake, better than auditory information, like 'get in the car we are going to get a milkshake'.

The assessment team will want to know what the child does when he wants or doesn't want something to understand how he expresses himself. Does he use adults like tools and take their hand and lead them to what he wants? Does he get agitated and distressed if he can't get what he wants for himself?

> For Siew, the team worked with Hong Yuan to ensure they had a clear understanding of what he understands in Mandarin as well as in English.

The assessment team needs to understand what communication skills each child has to develop communication strategies that are right for them.

> For Todd, who is verbal, the focus would be on the quality and content of his language and there are various language assessments which look at how children use language to express themselves and how much language they understand, both in terms of the meaning of words and the way words are combined in language. Todd's interpersonal communication or functional use of language and non-verbal communication would also be assessed. For example, can he take turns in a conversation? Does he know how to initiate and respond to greetings?

> The communication assessment for Jane would also include consideration of the communicative function of her behaviours. For example, when she screams is it to get attention, or is it because she isn't coping with a crowded noisy environment? Is she trying to 'tell' you something about what she is feeling or about her environment by her behaviour? This information is important because it will help the team, including Jane's family, identify alternative acceptable behaviours to be worked on with Jane.

DEVELOPMENTAL OR INTELLIGENCE ASSESSMENT

DSM-5 requires that for a child to be diagnosed with autism their social communication abilities must be below their other abilities. It is crucial therefore to understand your child's developmental stage and ability, and whether any of the behaviours are as expected for that stage. To assess your child's developmental ability, or if they are older, their intelligence, a standardised test will be administered. The test your child completes will depend on their age and observed abilities.

A developmental assessment provides useful information about your child's abilities in different areas such as balance, coordination and movement control, activities of self-care and independence, language, fine motor skills, visuospatial skills (the ability to visually perceive objects and the spatial relationships among objects), and the ability to solve practical problems and understand concepts. If your child has an intelligence test you will hear about their verbal and performance IQ based on their ability to understand, reason, identify relationships, problem-solve and process information. Both developmental and intelligence tests provide information about your child's abilities relative to children the same age. It is important to be aware that all tests measure specific skills in a certain way, and can only provide an assessment of performance on that day. As such, the results indicate the level of function your child achieved under the test conditions on that occasion. However, the types of tests used and the situation for testing is the sort that most children will face during the later preschool and school years. So even if the test results do not accurately reflect your child's ability, they are an indication of how they functioned in those circumstances, and that can be helpful information for planning intervention strategies and school placement. If your child did not engage during the assessment, it is possible that they will not engage in similar activities in school or other settings.

> Siew completed a developmental assessment. The paediatrician noted that in some areas of development, such as motor skills and visual skills, Siew was much better than in other areas like communication and social

development. She told Kenneth and Hong Yuan that on average Siew had a developmental age nearly two years behind his chronological age but that there was a lot of variability. For example, his communication and social development was equivalent to a typical child of twelve months, while his visuospatial skills were better than average for his age. She added that it wasn't clear how reliable the test results were because it was difficult to know if Siew failed to complete the tasks because he couldn't or because he wasn't interested, or because he was very stressed and anxious.

SENSORY PROBLEMS

Sensory problems are now included in the restricted and repetitive behaviour criteria for a diagnosis of autism, of which at least two behaviours must be present. An example is: 'Hyper- or hyporeactivity to sensory input or unusual interests in sensory aspects of the environment'.[5] In this sense, 'hyper' means oversensitive and 'hypo' means under-sensitive. Examples of sensory problems include: 'apparent indifference to pain/temperature, adverse response to specific or loud sounds or textures, excessive smelling or touching of objects, visual fascination with lights or movement'.[6] Indifference to pain or temperature would indicate hyporeactivity, while covering one's ears when exposed to loud sounds would indicate hyper-reactivity. As described in more detail in Chapter 6, it is not unusual for toddlers and preschool-aged children to have hyper- or hyporeactivity to some sensations, or indeed for it to persist into adulthood. The actual prevalence of sensory hyper- or hyporeactivity in the population is not known at different ages and estimates of the prevalence in autism also vary widely. While testing has failed to find any differences in the way people with autism hear sounds, people with autism who have hyper-reactive sound sensitivities report they frequently experience sounds as unpleasant or even as painful physiological sensations and may be fearful or anxious about hearing sounds as a result.

There are screening and assessment tools that can be used if sensory processing problems are suspected. These assess the sorts of behaviours that may result from sensory sensitivities and distortions, like holding hands over ears to block loud sounds, however we cannot at this stage measure sensory processing directly. This type of assessment can be useful for planning appropriate management strategies and should be used if you suspect your child has sensory problems or if your child has other behaviours that you think could be related to their sensory processing, like poor writing skills.

OTHER ASSESSMENTS THAT MAY BE HELPFUL

Following are other components of the assessment that may be helpful but are not required for making a diagnosis.

NEUROPSYCHOLOGY

There is still little proven about the key neuropsychological processes or information processing problems that are on the pathway to autism. However, depending on your child's presentation, assessments may be completed that will assess testable processes, such as working memory (the ability to hold and use information over short periods of time), executive function (forming a connection between past experience and present action in a way that helps us plan and organise), and theory of mind (the ability to infer from behaviours what others are thinking or feeling) to identify areas for intervention and to develop an understanding of some specific patterns of behaviour.

> Todd was seen by a neuropsychologist who identified that he had no concept that other people had thoughts and feelings different from his own, reflecting a delay in the development of theory of mind, which is usually

well developed by five years of age. She also noted that Todd had a poor working memory which, for example, made it difficult for him to recall complex directions (of more than two parts) he had just heard spoken by someone else.

TEMPERAMENT

We know that two children with autism can be as different as they are the same. Your child could be different from other children with autism because of the severity of their difficulties, or the specific autism behaviours they have, or because of other problems they do or don't have. In addition, your child's temperament is important both for their current management and their future planning. For example, children vary in the extent to which they persevere with a task or become frustrated; children may be outgoing and active or quiet and reflective. It is possible that the positive, or negative, attributes of your child's temperament will influence their experiences as much as the diagnosis of autism itself. It is important to take temperament and other personal attributes of your child into account when planning interventions and thinking about ways of maximising their strengths and potential.

> Jane had an active outgoing temperament and when faced with a noisy crowded situation she couldn't cope with, she was most likely to scream and lash out. Meanwhile, Todd was quieter and more withdrawn and in the same situation he responded by trying to get away to somewhere quiet.

MEDICAL INVESTIGATIONS

Not being able to hear or see will always affect the way we interact with our environment. All children who present with autism should have their hearing tested. This is not always straightforward but will be possible in a centre that is experienced with testing hearing in young children. If you have any concerns about your child's vision, that should also be formally tested.

It is generally accepted that genetic testing should be performed for all children diagnosed with autism. If your child also has an intellectual impairment they should have genetic testing for Fragile X. Modern genetic testing screens the genome, looking for differences to what is expected, and assesses any differences in relation to regions of DNA that are known to be associated with the types of problems your child has. If differences that could be relevant to autism behaviours or intellectual impairment are found, then genetic testing will be carried out on the biological parents to identify if the difference was passed from one or both parents or has occurred for the first time in your child. This can be a useful test for finding whether there is a risk that a difference could be present in other children you have. Your child's test results may also add to our broader understanding of the genetic causes of autism.

Note that there is a difference between general genetic tests and genetic discoveries from research. Genes are increasingly being identified in research as being associated with autism. However, at the time of writing, there is insufficient strong evidence of a direct cause from specific genes to recommend specific gene testing. The Simons Foundation Autism Research Initiative (or SFARI) has a website (see Resources at the end of this chapter) that is listing candidate genes as they are reported with a rating of evidence for their causal role. It also lists genes linked to known syndromes in which autism occurs.

Other medical investigations ordered for your child will depend on the type of problems that they have. If they have funny turns that could be seizures or if they are known to have had one or more seizures when they did not have a fever, an electroencephalogram, usually known as an EEG and which provides information about electrical brain activity, may be ordered.

Brain imaging, usually performed using magnetic resonance imaging (known as an MRI) might also be ordered if your child has any problems that suggest parts of the nervous system other than those usually affected by autism could be causing some of their problems.

This would be done, for example, for some types of seizures, as for John, or if there are problems with motor skills.

> John had an EEG as he had a seizure when he did not have a fever. An assessment of his ability identified that he had a severe intellectual disability as well as autism. When his seizures were difficult to control with single agent medication, his epilepsy specialist and developmental paediatrician decided that neuroimaging, using MRI, should also be done. John had a general anaesthetic to make sure he was still for the MRI. No problem with the structure of his brain was found.

If on examination your child has any other finding that suggests a physical illness, then investigations will be tailored to explore the possible causes and implications. For example, if they are a fussy eater (see also Chapter 6) and have been irritable or lethargic, then blood tests could be ordered to look for anaemia, either due to an iron, vitamin B_{12} or folate deficiency. If they are known to eat things that could contain lead, then lead levels will be tested.

IF SKILLS ARE LOST

The toddler years, when skill loss is most commonly reported, is a difficult time to assess development and, as such, a difficult time to assess if skills have plateaued, gained slightly or decreased. There are some helpful definitions of skill loss but in brief a skill should have been present for at least a couple of months and then absent for at least a couple of months before it is considered to have been lost.

> Todd's presentation is reported in a minority of children with autism with a loss of early words and observation of distress during social interaction. Todd was using one- to two-word phrases at eighteen months but

language development stalled and between eighteen and 24 months he stopped using these early words. He also became very quiet and avoided interaction with people around him although he liked to be close to Jessica and Joseph and became very distressed if one of them was not close by.

Siew had a similar history but with co-occurring major social change. He had started to talk (Mandarin) when he was eighteen months old and was very attached to his grandmother in Singapore, but when the family moved to Australia he stopped talking and became quite withdrawn and distant. By then Hong Yuan was pregnant with Leila, who was born three months after Hong Yuan and Kenneth arrived in Australia, and because the family had just moved countries and cultures they felt this might be distressing Siew.

The reason for interest in skill loss is that it can indicate an underlying biological problem that could require a different form of examination, investigation and, depending on what is found, intervention. A paediatrician is the right professional to assist with the assessment that is needed to identify if there is a known underlying biological cause.

Loss of skills, also known as developmental regression, was first described in autism in the 1960s. Many theories exist about the cause of the observed skill loss and behaviour change that is seen in autism, but none have yet been proven.

Not all children who present with skill loss and problems of the type seen in autism have an underlying biological problem identified, but this is one of those instances where it is important to rule out possible causes. The types of tests a paediatrician could recommend include specific genetic testing, for example looking for the Rett gene in girls with autism, and also some mentioned earlier, like MRI and EEG, but are not limited to these. An EEG is useful for identifying seizure disorders, some of which may not be obvious because they do not cause collapse or jerking movements. These tests, except for an examination of your child's DNA, are only ordered if there is a loss of skills or some other reason for concern, such as poor diet or a problem with movement, muscle strength or muscle tone.

> Todd gradually made language gains and at five years he was speaking using two- to three-word phrases. Todd's subsequent language development ruled out the more severe biological causes of skill loss.

> The changes in Siew's development, with loss of skills, were noticed at the same time that substantial changes occurred in his and his family's life. It was thought that the social changes that were occurring had made Siew stressed or anxious and that this had caused a short-term failure to use acquired skills or that unwanted behaviours had replaced positive ones. However, possible biological causes for skill loss were investigated and he was monitored to ensure he didn't have ongoing skill loss.

DIFFERENT TYPES OF AUTISM

Different types of autism are no longer defined by *DSM-5*. Instead, the type of autism is described by the other diagnoses that your child may or may not have, such as intellectual disability, attention deficit hyperactivity disorder or specific language impairment (SLI), sometimes described as language learning impairment. Or your child's type of autism might be identified because of their path to the problems they have, either because they are known to have a genetic problem, like Fragile X or tuberous sclerosis, or a seizure disorder from early life, like John. The *DSM-5* severity levels, described earlier, can also be used to identify different types of autism. If Jane, Todd, Siew and John were diagnosed using *DSM-5* criteria we would have the following additional information.

> Jane would have been diagnosed as autism spectrum disorder with a Level 2, 'requiring substantial support' severity level for both the social communication and restricted and repetitive behaviours categories. She would be described as having borderline intellectual impairment and accompanying language impairment.

> Todd would have been diagnosed as autism spectrum disorder with accompanying language impairment, without accompanying intellectual impairment. Todd's severity for social communication problems and restricted repetitive behaviours would both be Level 1, 'requiring support'.

> Siew would have been diagnosed as autism spectrum disorder with accompanying language impairment and mild intellectual disability. Siew's ASD severity level would have been assessed as Level 3, 'requiring very substantial support' for social communication and as Level 1, 'requiring support' for restricted repetitive behaviours.

> John would have been diagnosed as autism spectrum disorder, with accompanying intellectual disability and a severity score for social communication of Level 3, 'requiring very substantial support' and for restricted and repetitive behaviours of Level 2, 'requiring substantial support'.

This way of thinking about different types of autism is often referred to as a dimensional approach, and provides the advantage of including important information so professionals can understand your child's particular difficulties, abilities and needs. It also creates a framework for research because more specific diagnoses are helpful in advancing interventions and causal discoveries. But most importantly, it creates an individual picture of your child that will be helpful for developing their individual therapy (see Chapter 5) and educational plans (see chapters 7 and 9). As their learning patterns and difficulties abilities change, the diagnosis, severity scores and specifiers will need to be reviewed and can continue to provide nuanced information that can assist longer term planning for your child and the rest of your family.

WHAT HAPPENS NEXT?

First, make sure you understand everything that has been discussed with you by the assessment team. If you disagree with aspects of the assessment, can't understand some of the information that has been presented, or are dissatisfied with how the process was completed, go back to the team you saw and ask for clarification and advice or tell them you are unhappy with the process. Unless you do this the team or individuals you have been working with will not know you have concerns that have not been addressed. Remember that exchanges — whether face-to-face, over the phone or by email — are more likely to be successful if you are calm and composed. If you feel unable to ask about what you want to know without becoming emotional, then it is quite reasonable to ask a friend or family member to help you.

Next, make sure you know what services are planned for your child. If anything is unclear, go back to the assessment team and get more information about the possible next steps, any options that are available, how long it should be before you hear from somebody and what you need to do. You'll be trying to make sure your child gets all the assistance they need, so don't be afraid to ask questions and remember, service providers base their decisions on the information you give them, so make sure you tell it like it is. The types of things that could be useful are discussed further in chapters 5 and 7.

Finally, every parent feels differently following an assessment and diagnosis of autism. The professionals you are working with will understand that receiving a diagnosis can be a very stressful and challenging time. It is all right to ask for assistance for yourself and other family members as you make necessary changes and come to understand what this means for you and your child.

RESOURCES

Autism spectrum disorder criteria

See Resources in Chapter 1

Different diagnostic tests that can be used

http://onlinelibrary.wiley.com/doi/10.1002/14651858.CD009044/abstract

Types of genetic tests explained further

https://sfari.org/news-and-opinion/news/2010/microarray-analysis-deemed-best-genetic-test-for-autism

www.gsnv.org.au/media/223085/microarray_factsheet_gsnv_vcgs.pdf

Up-to-date information on research findings about genetic causes

https://gene.sfari.org/autdb/GS_Home.do

Information from research about loss of skills or regression

http://sfari.org/news-and-opinion/news/2012/regression-may-mark-one-third-of-autism-cases

Up-to-date guidelines for a diagnosis of autism

www.nice.org.uk/guidance/cg128 for access to all elements of the guidelines or http://pathways.nice.org.uk/pathways/autism for the recommended pathway.

www.health.govt.nz/our-work/disability-services/disability-projects-and-programmes/autism-spectrum-disorder-guideline

www.waadf.org.au/WAADF_ASD_Assessment_Process_2012.pdf

www.amaze.org.au/discover/about-autism-spectrum-disorder/assessment-diagnosis/ and for more detail www.amaze.org.au/uploads/2013/06/ASD-Diagnosis-Assessment-Guidelines-Victoria-2009.pdf

www.asha.org/policy/GL2006-00049.htm

www.autism.org.uk/about-autism/all-about-diagnosis.aspx

CHAPTER 4

LOOKING AFTER YOURSELF

Autism doesn't just affect the child who has been diagnosed — it affects the whole family. You need to be physically and emotionally well to support your child with autism, the other people you love and to participate in the community or the workplace as you choose.

An important part of looking after yourself is making sure you are not hard on yourself. Most parents wonder if they are to blame for the problems that their child has. In this chapter, we talk about why you might be wondering if you are to blame, and why you actually aren't. We also provide some ideas of ways to look after yourself.

DID I CAUSE THIS?

'Did I cause this?' is one of the questions that parents of a child who has developmental problems will often ask themselves. You may never voice the question openly, but if you do, you will likely find you get a different answer on different days from different people.

There are some important things to consider with this issue. Modern thinking leads us to believe that we are able to control, or at least influence, most things in our life. We hear this every day in multiple ways and can start to feel that, if we make the right choices, we will be able to avoid any problems altogether. Most people living in high-income countries have more choice today than ever before. However, you don't need to have worked in health, education or disability care for long to realise that many things happen over which we have no control.

Parents of children with autism are particularly likely to ask questions about their role in possible causes. This may be because autism was historically embedded in psychiatry. Theories about styles of mothering (such as so-called 'refrigerator mothers') have been an important, but now discredited, part of the condition's history. It may be because the problems seen in autism are not physical, as with cerebral palsy, or easily measured or described, like a speech (articulation) disorder, that they appear more open to influence.

It is also possible that once your child has been identified as having difficulties, you will review every event up to the time their problems began, thoroughly and often.

> Many mothers have a birth history very similar to the one shared by Jane and Todd, with a long labour culminating in a caesarean section. That history alone would not suggest any possible cause of Todd's problems, but Jessica is likely to have pondered those events more often than a mother whose child is developing without concerns.

Scientists may be unwittingly compounding feelings that you have caused your child to have autism. Today, researchers are encouraged to be visible and to communicate science with the public. This can lead to theories about the causes of conditions like autism becoming widely available before they are proven, and before any work has been completed to decide if the theories are helpful for children and their families. For what to look for when assessing information about possible causes of autism see Chapter 11. There are also an increasing number of blogs online that are being written by people trained to look at science with skepticism, some of whom also have children with autism. Some of these are listed in the Resources at the end of the chapter.

The rise in health care initiatives that focus on prevention has also led to an expectation that there may be some way of preventing autism. There are some diseases and problems that we know are preventable and science and health care are always keen to follow the proverb 'prevention is better than cure' where possible. Not surprisingly, the brain is an area where less is known about how to prevent problems, and autism is one of the most complex disorders of the brain. Currently, there is no high quality evidence identifying potentially preventable causes of autism that would have been within your control.

SHOULD I HAVE REALISED EARLIER?

This is another question that you may be asking, while feeling guilty that opportunities for interventions have been missed. It is true that everything is always clearer with hindsight. In medicine, this is thought of as looking at things with the 'retrospectoscope'. With the 'retrospectoscope' it is always clear what should have been done.

When you look back at your child's early life, it is likely that there were behaviours that you now think were markers of autism. Take, for example, Jane's sleeping and eating patterns when she was an infant and toddler.

> Jane was a restless baby and difficult to soothe. She would wriggle and scream when Louise tried to hold her and only slept for a few hours at a time. Louise was exhausted much of the time trying to manage Jane as well as care for her other children. Jane was difficult to

feed, she refused the breast and it took a long time to feed her with a bottle as she was easily distracted.

But many children will exhibit those behaviours during the first and second year of life and if they resolve and no other problems occur their parents will give them little further thought. Even some behaviours more often linked to autism, like arm flapping when excited or anxious, a lack of interest in others, and covering ears and screaming when there are loud sounds, occur in children who do not have continued problems of the type seen in autism.

> Many children are placid as babies like Siew was. Others are like his younger sister who, when she was a few months old, cooed and gurgled, smiled and clearly sought and responded to her family. Those differences would not have been relevant or meaningful if Siew was now making good developmental gains.

Trained and experienced professionals also have problems accurately identifying autism early in life. Even a multidisciplinary assessment team involving doctors, psychologists and speech therapists will not be perfect at correctly identifying those children who will have developmental problems. Why is this? Children under twelve months of age have limited ways to communicate their basic needs, such as food, nappy changes and sleep. Between six and twelve months of age children develop more clearly their likes and dislikes, need for attention and identify very strongly with their main caregivers, but still have a limited range of ways to communicate their thoughts and feelings. Between one and two years of age the ability to communicate increases. There are many developmental gains during this second twelve months with emerging physical, emotional, social, communication and reasoning skills, but not all children make these gains in the same sequence or in the same way, and temperament can change these behaviours as well.

There are many varied patterns of human development in early life which means it is not always possible to tell which ones will lead to problems in understanding, learning, and social communication, or restricted and repetitive behaviours, sensory problems and a lack of interest in others. For example, some children learn language first and other things follow, others master practical reasoning before language and communication. Some make relatively smooth developmental gains but most have plateaus and then developmentally 'take-off' intermittently. Most can't learn multiple things at once. This variation in development means that behaviours that occur at one point in time are not necessarily predictive of what happens next. So to know if something is going to be a problem, we have to see what happens next.

WHEN CAN WE FIRST IDENTIFY AUTISM?

Opinions vary about the age at which children with autism can accurately be diagnosed, and there are different practices and expectations in different countries. Most children who are found to have autism are currently diagnosed after the age of two and before the end of primary school, using the behavioural methods described in Chapter 3.

Until recently, little has been known about how children with and without autism differ from each other during the first year of life, or about signs that may assist with early identification or diagnosis. The most recent information has come from sibling studies that have investigated the behaviour of babies who are known to have a brother or sister with autism. These studies have so far shown no difference in developmental pathways toward either autism or normal development and no single behaviour or test result has been identified that would correctly identify all children with autism before the age of one. Between the ages of one and two, more behaviours have been reported to show a change in the rate of development that are linked to a later diagnosis of autism, including problems with shared attention, social interest and language use. However, findings have differed between studies in relation to the behaviours seen. Remembering that these are studies that are conducted from early life with regular reviews and follow-ups until the age of three when a diagnosis is made using some highly sophisticated tests, it is not surprising that most parents do not have concerns before the age of two.

IT'S NEVER TOO LATE TO LEARN

You may have heard intervention is more effective early on and that if you don't start early you will not get results. Even if your child's autism was not identified at a young age, you shouldn't worry. While it may be easier to learn some skills when young, such as a musical instrument or another language, there are some things that require other developmental and learning foundations to be in place before they can be mastered. This is why most children don't learn advanced mathematics in primary school. We also know that with some tasks that can be learnt at a young age, older children quickly reach the same level even if they start later. Music is a common example. So the saying 'It is never too late to learn' applies here. Learning is an incremental process during which we build on success. We are all life-long learners. When thinking about your child's learning capabilities, think about their current strengths and difficulties, and about interventions that are appropriate to their needs and abilities now. You need to be ready for the intervention too, and it has to be the best thing for the whole of your family. So if you didn't realise your child had autism in the first years of life, don't worry. There are still many opportunities for learning.

BE KIND TO YOURSELF

Being a parent is very tiring. There are both physical and emotional challenges, often at the same time, such as chasing your child to bring them back from a dangerous place. Some difficult behaviours can also go on for a long time, such as a tantrum in a supermarket where passers-by start to offer advice, make comments about you as a parent, or appear to be silently judging you. Yet during this stressful time, you need to be in charge, consistent in your approach and readily available for your child.

If that is the lot of any parent or carer, what does that mean for you? There is no doubt that you will face additional challenges in day-to-day activities. You will also be trying to accept that your child is different from the one you expected. You may also have been feeling guilty because you thought you caused this, or that you didn't recognise that your child had autism soon enough. You may also feel as though you aren't helping your child enough. You may even feel pressured by other parents to try interventions and strategies they are convinced worked for their children and be made to feel guilty if you decide not to do so. There are so many ways that you hear about helping your child, but you can't do all of them.

> Remember John's mother Sue. The mothers in the support group were trying lots of different therapies and interventions and some of them were convinced that their child was allergic to wheat and dairy and this was the cause of their autism. Sue felt she should try this diet with John but worried about how it would fit in with the rest of the family.

So how in amongst all that can you look after yourself? Different people cope in different ways and there is definitely no 'one size fits all'. Usually, any given individual uses more than one way to cope with stress. Remember, it is particularly important that you get enough sleep, regular physical activity and that you eat nutritious, well-balanced meals. You also need breaks from caring for your child with autism to ensure you get time to relax, socialise and do some of the activities you enjoy.

Feeling well supported is important. It is fine to ask for help. You can seek support from parents, friends, and family, but problems can arise if you rely on those closest to you as your sole source of support. You can also seek support from your child's professionals and your local doctor.

If they are not able to assist they will know of other professionals who can. Some parents gain enormous strength from parents' groups, while others find they cause more problems than they resolve. This is a very personal decision.

> Sue, John's mum, found it very hard to talk to her friends about what was happening with John and her family; their experiences with their own young children were so different from her own and when she tried taking John with her to visit them and play with their children she found John became very distressed. He avoided being with other children, especially when they were noisy, and would find a quiet place by himself and some books to flip through. Sue pushed John to join in with the other children but he became very agitated and distressed and would make loud angry noises and take her hand and pull her towards the door. John was clearly very different from the other children. Her friends were sympathetic but had very little understanding of her situation and invited her and John over less and less often. Sue joined a parent support group and found that being with other women in the same situation as herself was a great help. She would have liked Mike to come as well but the group met one morning a week when he was at work. Besides, there were no other fathers in the group and Sue knew Mike would be uncomfortable in an all-female group. The parent support group started to organise family outings together at the weekends. Mike came sometimes but Sam, John's brother, usually chose to spend time with his friends from school.

Along the way it is good to acknowledge that you and others close to you may cope quite differently. It is also important to acknowledge that, although well-meaning, not all advice is good advice. You are in charge of the decisions about your child and even though advice can be heeded, it does not always have to be followed.

For Hong Yuan and Kenneth, Siew's parents, they had a live-in grandmother, Zhen Zhu, who flatly refused to accept anything was wrong with Siew while at the same time telling them to take him to China for some traditional medicine. This difference of opinion created tension between Kenneth and Zhen Zhu.

This sort of situation can cause conflict, not only with the person providing the well-meaning advice but also between parents. It is important to acknowledge this sort of situation as it arises and for parents to confer to ensure they agree about the best way to manage the situation.

Learning more about yourself and how you cope in stressful situations may be helpful. Early on as a parent it is worth identifying what your own strengths and limitations are in terms of managing yourself and your child. This makes calling in assistance as needed much more straightforward if problems arise.

Many parents also enjoy working and the different environment and challenges that brings, while others find working an added stress. Having a child with autism may create barriers to returning to work that other parents do not face. For example, finding satisfactory child care can be more difficult. Or you may need to work closer to your child care or school because you are being asked to attend the school more frequently to consult with the staff.

Sue, John's mum, wanted to return to some part-time work once John and his older brother Sam were at school each day but that was hard for her, not only because John had autism. Jobs were hard to find in the outer suburbs where the family lived and the family could only afford one car which John's Dad, Mike, drove each day to his work as a mechanic, so Sue had to rely on the infrequent local bus service during the day.

You may also find that you feel differently than you expected about going back to work. You could be experiencing feelings of guilt because of your new view of your expected role as parent of a child with additional needs, one who needs to be available to attend early intervention for example, or because of the way you feel others think about your role, expecting you to be managing your child constantly. You could be feeling anxious because of the added pressure for you and your family that working will bring. Returning to work is not a simple decision for parents and it needs to take into account many factors. But it is not a decision you should avoid either. Think through the advantages and disadvantages of returning to work and make sure you put your own wellbeing into the decision-making equation (see Resources at the end of this chapter).

SUPPORTING PARENTING AND PROBLEM-SOLVING

There are many different parenting programs that are available today designed to teach parents useful strategies to manage problem behaviours in young children. Some are for parents of children with autism and are often linked to an early intervention program, while others are used more widely (see Resources at the end of this chapter). These programs usually share approaches to parenting preschool-aged children, including being consistent in your expectations and setting reasonable limits or boundaries. Most report positive outcomes for parents as well as improvements in child behaviour.

Established interventions for parents of older children either work with parents alone or with parents and young people together and adopt problem-solving approaches. These types of programs can be useful in preventing future problems, but availability can vary depending on where you live. Your local community health service, early intervention team or local doctor should know what is available close to you.

WHEN THE USUAL THINGS YOU DO AND FRIENDS AND FAMILY AREN'T ENOUGH

For some of you, watching your child have difficulties or being told that they have autism will cause you to reflect on your own behaviours more than other parents might, and you may also reflect on your own childhood.

> Todd's mother, Jessica, realised that many of her problems could be because she had similar behaviours and ways of thinking to Todd. She knew she was highly intelligent and focused and in her area of expertise she was recognised internationally. However, she also realised that her academic career had been patchy, and despite her considerable ability and intellect her applications for promotion had been unsuccessful. Jessica felt that she had never quite understood how the system worked and often found herself offending people without understanding why. She admitted that she had blamed others for her lack of professional advancement before she understood about autism. When she was diagnosed with Asperger's disorder she felt relief. Jessica wanted to go back to work once Todd was going to school but the team she worked with before she went on maternity leave had since moved on and Jessica was very anxious about working with different people who didn't know her.

Other ways you cope with stress may also become more apparent to you, or you may realise that although you had behaviours and methods of coping that worked for you before, they are not helping now that you have additional responsibilities. Similarly, coping strategies, like respite with grandparents, may be less available because your child has autism.

> Todd's grandparents live close by, however they believe his problems are a result of him being with his mother constantly and being 'babied'. So although Todd stays with them from time to time, his visits usually end with them bringing him home early very distressed because they get annoyed when he repeatedly asks questions about what will happen next, which he does more often when his routine changes.

Apart from the physical burden of care this creates there is also the added emotional burden that family conflict and being judged brings.

Approaches to promote mental wellbeing are becoming increasingly available. Some are also effective as interventions when problems arise. For example, mindfulness and acceptance and commitment therapy (ACT) may provide approaches that you find useful to assist you to cope with any distress or stress you are experiencing. These are relatively recent models of psychotherapy, with some common underpinnings to meditation that are also known as 'third wave' or a 'new generation' of psychological therapies. Emerging, but not yet high quality, evidence (see Chapter 10 for more about how to work out what is high quality evidence) suggests that these types of interventions are just as effective as more traditional forms of cognitive and behavioural therapies for treating depression and may be useful for reducing anxiety and distress (see Resources at the end of this chapter). Your local doctor will know how to find and access services that promote mental wellbeing for you.

Adult mental health services accessed via your local doctor, including psychiatrists, psychologists, social workers or mental health nurses, are an excellent resource for personal, relationship or family counselling and can help you make decisions about whether further intervention is needed, and the most appropriate type of intervention for your current situation and difficulties. When it comes to your health, and in particular mental health, the best approach is to ask for help if you are experiencing distress, feel very stressed or very sad. Also ask for help if you have persistent low energy and mood or if others are telling you they are worried about you and your behaviour. Professionals do not need to see your best performance at being happy and coping. They need to hear and see the real issues so they can assist you. It is definitely okay to seek help for yourself. This is not taking attention away from the important needs of your child or in any way detracting from their best care. In fact, quite the opposite. Thinking about yourself and what you need and seeking assistance when it is needed will help your child or young person with autism as much as it helps you, and the rest of your family. Investing in yourself so you feel rested, resilient and able to cope is incredibly important. Do it whenever and however you can.

SIBLINGS

Your other children will need some help understanding that their brother or sister has autism, and what that means for you and them. When you are busy with your child with autism, your other children may miss out on your time and attention, which may lead to feelings of resentment. They may also be worried about how to tell their friends that their brother or sister has autism, and whether they can still bring friends home. These issues will need to be addressed.

Much of the information they need will be similar to the information you find helpful, adapted for their age. Be open and honest with your other children about what having autism means and communicate to them what changes will take place in the family home. Let them know how they can assist their brother or sister and also how they can assist you. Make the ways they help both doable and rewarding. Keep in mind that playing an active part in family life is different to taking on a role as their sibling's carer. Both will give them life skills but the latter comes with responsibilities that may have negative impacts too. There are support groups for siblings that some, but not all, will find helpful. There is an increasing amount of material, including books and films, about the experiences of siblings of a child with a disability, and specifically with autism, as well as some helpful web-based resources. Talk openly about how others think about children and adults with additional needs so they are forewarned about comments they may hear and behaviours they may see. And remember, they also need to spend time with you so try to plan activities with them so they feel valued too (see Resources at the end of this chapter).

> Jane's brother and sister, Jade and Hayden, were included in the team to plan and manage her program at secondary school. This helped them to understand the things that were difficult for Jane and how to help. At first Hayden didn't want to know but when his friends found out how good Jane was at computer games he started to enjoy showing off about his sister. Jade and her friends began to watch out for Jane, especially when other students tried to tease or bully her. The school made sure that Jade and Hayden were acknowledged for their role in supporting Jane and received lots of positive feedback. As a result, family relationships improved at home and Louise found she was able to take all three of her children out together.

RESOURCES

Comments on early identification and intervention

www.ncbi.nlm.nih.gov/pmc/articles/PMC3913013/

http://informahealthcare.com/doi/full/10.3109/17549507.2013.859732

http://informahealthcare.com/doi/full/10.3109/17549507.2013.859300

http://informahealthcare.com/doi/full/10.3109/17549507.2013.861870

http://raisingchildren.net.au/articles/autism_spectrum_disorder_early_signs.html

Review of findings for early predictors of autism from prospective longitudinal studies

www.ncbi.nlm.nih.gov/pmc/articles/PMC3969297/

Approaches to looking after yourself

www.ndis.gov.au/sites/default/files/documents/Wellbeing%20Resource.pdf

www.autism-help.org/family-autism-self-care-strategies.htm

Psychological interventions for parents of children and adolescents with chronic illness

http://onlinelibrary.wiley.com/doi/10.1002/14651858.CD009660.pub2/abstract

http://ps.psychiatryonline.org/article.aspx?articleID=1730565

Systematic reviews of 'third wave' cognitive and behavioural therapies for depression or anxiety

http://onlinelibrary.wiley.com/doi/10.1002/14651858.CD008704.pub2/abstract;jsessionid=A65521DDCB3A874643B9434E383C26F3.f04t04

www.ncbi.nlm.nih.gov/pmc/articles/PMC2848393/

Siblings

http://raisingchildren.net.au/articles/autism_spectrum_disorder_siblings.html

www.autism.org.uk/about-autism/all-about-diagnosis/diagnosis-the-process-for-children/recently-diagnosed-children.aspx

CHAPTER 5

THE TODDLER AND PRESCHOOL YEARS

In this chapter we present the main features of encouraging communication and managing the behaviour of a toddler or pre-school-aged child with autism, as well as information about early interventions, mainly based on learning. These approaches can be used from the toddler and preschool years onward and are key to managing any specific problems that may arise (see also chapters 6, 7, 8 and 9).

During the toddler and preschool years your child will spend more time with you than at any other stage. It is hard to say what each child with autism experiences of the people in their world. We do know that having a small number of important people in the early years of life is one of the foundations for future development and wellbeing. The fact that you're there for your child, that you care about them and are providing a safe environment with opportunities to learn is important, even if your child doesn't respond in the way you expect. Whether or not you are receiving positive feedback, assume your child will know that you love them.

The toddler years (one- to two-year-olds) pose unique issues for parents. These are the years before language is well developed which means behaviours are harder to anticipate and seem unpredictable. They are also the years during which children are very active and where there is action without understanding or concern for risk, which leads to high physical demands on parents who need to be watching — or chasing — their children all the time. These are also the years where a child and family are likely to get into struggles about who is in charge, adding to the physical and emotional demands on parents or carers. These years are also the most challenging for gathering information about development because we can't access what your child is feeling or thinking. Rather, we rely on observing behaviour, which can be highly variable from child to child and even in one child on different days in different places (see Resources at the end of this chapter).

For children with autism the problems with social communication and restricted or repetitive behaviours, including resistance to change, add to the physical and emotional load of parenting. Also for children with autism, the phase in which it is hard to know what your child is thinking can be prolonged, as can be some of the more negative 'toddler' behaviours.

The preschool years (three- to four-year-olds) mark an important developmental progression with increased social communication and the ability to separate from parents and well-known carers. During the preschool years children show an increased interest in other people, and peers in particular. Autism is commonly diagnosed at this age due to a lack of expected developmental progress. This is the age in which social communication skills develop rapidly in most children. Preschool children also gain confidence in their ability to manage themselves and generally thrive on being given opportunities, within their ability level, to assist others and organise their environment. During the preschool years children start to verbalise their curiosity as questions, sometimes asked repeatedly. Children of this age still enjoy routines and benefit from knowing they have consistency and constancy in carers. Their ability to take turns grows and consolidates during these years (see Resources at the end of this chapter).

Developing readiness for school is an important part of the preschool years. This requires developmental or cognitive abilities, social abilities and also emotional regulation. During these years you'll be thinking about helping your child to develop these skills and also about the right school for your child.

During the toddler and preschool years it is easy to worry about the things your child is having difficulties with because you will spend a lot of time with them. However, it is good to also consider your child's strengths and whether there are ways to use these to further develop areas in which they are having difficulty. During these years you know your child better than anyone else, and your insights into their strengths and needs are very important.

Although they may seem too young to understand during these years, your child will know when you are stressed or if there have been major events in your life, like the death of a parent, separation or a new baby. Such events are likely to change your child's mood, behaviour or both. Seek help for yourself and also advice about how to best communicate any problems or changes with your child. Additional assistance at times like these can be invaluable.

This is also the age when children work out how to press your buttons to get a reaction, both positive and negative. They learn how to press their brothers' and sisters' buttons too. You need to know this so you can identify it when it is happening. It's also the age when consistency in the way you respond is very important.

Managing behaviour requires good communication and is an integral part of learning so, in practice, managing behaviour, communication and learning are intertwined with gains in one area linked to improvements in others. Communication failure underpins many problem behaviours, so if we start with understanding and improving communication, we are likely to find problem behaviours are reduced and learning is enhanced.

ENCOURAGING COMMUNICATION

Communication is an integral part of all behaviour and learning, so working on enhancing your child's ability to express themselves and to understand language should be a high priority. Speech therapists are communication experts. They are trained to identify speech and language abilities and difficulties, to promote speech, language and social communication development (such as turn-taking), and to teach your child strategies to aid communication.

Long before children start to speak they are engaging and communicating with others using eye contact, sounds and gestures. Other early social communication behaviours include the imitation of movements, actions or sounds and shared attention (often called joint attention), when your child shows you something using eye contact or gesture and responds to your attempts to show them something by looking at you and at what you are showing them.

Your child may respond to bids for shared attention less than most children do and may rarely initiate shared attention by showing you something. Your child may be less interested in or unable to imitate the movement and actions of others, although as they develop and start to speak they may have excellent verbal imitation skills (echolalia). We don't know why this discrepancy between motor and verbal imitation occurs.

Engagement, shared attention and imitation are all essential for the development of language and slowness or lack of development in these areas often indicates delayed or disordered language and social development. What can we do to improve social communication development? The key is to focus on engagement.

Siew's speech therapist worked with Siew each week at the clinic and also with Hong Yuan and Kenneth and with the staff at the playgroup to set up a communication program for him. She focused first of all on engaging Siew, playing games he liked which involved taking turns, and setting up the clinic room so that he had to communicate with her to get what he wanted.

Your child may process and remember information they see better than information they hear. When they see static visual information they can take as long as they need to process it compared to hearing information which is only there for as long as it takes to say. This is why visual supports are useful to enable your child to communicate, learn, process information, and manage their physical and social environment. Motivation is also very important. Your child is most likely to learn to communicate with you about things and activities they really like.

> Siew's speech therapist noted that Siew liked DVDs, books, musical instruments, push-down toys, action–response toys and 'peek-a-boo' games. He flapped his hands and smiled when a carer made a noise with a toy. She paired spoken words for his favourite things and activities with photos and drawings and taught him to give her the picture of what he wanted. She worked with the playgroup staff and with Hong Yuan to do the same at home and in the group.

A number of communication-focused interventions are used which capitalise on relatively good visual information processing skills which, in turn, compensates for difficulties with understanding what is said. These interventions are most effective when they are integrated into an early intervention program that also includes other elements. The term 'augmentative and alternative communication' (AAC) is used for many of these strategies and includes the use of real objects, picture symbols, manual signing, and speech-generating devices to support both what your child wants to communicate and what you want to communicate to your child.

> Siew didn't imitate words or sounds but sometimes reached out and placed his hand on a toy. He demonstrated some understanding of real objects and

photos, and responded to one-word verbal prompts to indicate 'come' and hand gestures to wave 'bye'.

Zhen Zhu, Siew's grandmother, protested because she thought if he learnt to use pictures and gestures to communicate he would never start talking again but she did find it useful herself to have a way of communicating with him. The pictures always had the word printed underneath in Mandarin and in English which she found helped her learn some basic English words. Siew responded really well to the program and communicated more often and more reliably with key people around him. He started to repeat the spoken words he heard, sometimes in English, sometimes in Mandarin. He also started to draw the words and clearly had an excellent memory for written words in both languages. He liked to go over the daily routine with his mother in the morning looking at a picture schedule for the day and liked to take the pictures and put them in the 'finished' envelope as activities were completed.

It is important to work out exactly how, why, when and with whom your child communicates as this is your starting point. Remember communication is the key, not speech. There are some useful resources to help you work out what communication skills your child has and therefore where to start focusing on developing their communication. For example, The Pragmatics Profile of Everyday Communication Skills in Children is a useful assessment for functional communication (also called pragmatics). It is free of charge (see Resources at the end of this chapter).

Many parents who are bilingual worry about whether they should speak only one language to simplify language learning for their child, when they find that their child is having difficulties learning to communicate. Each family and child is different, so the right solution for one family may not be the same for another. What we do know is that the focus should always be on communication and engagement and communication is most effective in the first language of family members. If families are using another language to communicate with their child, the quality and frequency of their interactions are likely to be affected. Also, if a child does not learn their family's first language, then their ability to communicate with their family and community will be compromised, as will their understanding of their family's culture. There is no evidence to suggest that children with autism have more difficulty learning language if one language (e.g. Mandarin) is spoken at home and another (e.g. English) is spoken at preschool. The difficulties they have are primarily with the use or function of language and this difficulty is consistent in monolingual and bilingual situations.

> Siew's parents, Hong Yuan and Kenneth, debated the advantages of having their children grow up bilingual. They felt that perhaps just speaking English, the language of their adopted country, would reduce the burden on Siew. In the end they made a pragmatic decision and continued as a bilingual household to cater for Zhen Zhu as well as their desire to equip their children with both Mandarin and English.

MANAGING BEHAVIOUR

Our capacity to cope with situations we find difficult and stressful is called resilience. Children with autism are coping with a world they find bewildering and challenging and find themselves in more situations that are difficult or stressful than their peers. We need to find ways of increasing their resilience so they will be able to cope with unexpected and novel situations as well as situations that are known to be difficult or stressful. We can also manage the environment to reduce the challenges experienced. For example, we can increase the predicability and routine of activities and present information visually. Stressed and anxious children learn less, so developing strategies for them to cope in situations that can't be minimised or avoided is important and will build resilience as well.

For children with autism, unwanted behaviours may be an attempt to communicate, or may stem from trying to cope with a situation that is stressful, like a change of route on the way home or a change in activities. We refer to this as the 'communicative function' of the behaviour, which may be intentional, that is, your child is trying to tell you what they want but doesn't know how to do this in an acceptable way (like pushing you to the fridge when they want a drink) or it may be unintentional, where your child is acting or reacting to something in the environment (like screaming and throwing food if you serve them a different meal).

Behaviour does not occur in a vacuum, and almost always has an antecedent (also called a trigger), a purpose (a function), and a consequence. It is essential to understand why a behaviour occurs, what triggers it, and what maintains it, if we are to have any hope of changing it. This is known as the A–B–C of behaviour (Antecedent–Behaviour–Consequence) (see Resources at the end of this chapter).

Triggers for unwanted behaviours can vary widely and include being provoked by another child, an unexpected change or a physical problem. Your child may have communication problems that make it difficult for them to tell you if they are sick or in pain. Your child may also have unusual responses to pain or discomfort and may under- or over-react or react in a way that does not identify the problem. So if your child's behaviour changes substantially and relatively suddenly, it is important to consider whether any physical or health problems could be causing the change and to seek help from your doctor. Also think about whether the problem could be dental, like a tooth abscess, because your child may attend the dentist less frequently than other children because of the difficulties experienced during dental appointments.

Working out the function of an unwanted behaviour for your child is important. Sometimes this isn't obvious and it takes some detective work and lateral thinking to figure out; at other times it is very clear. The function of the behaviour could include getting something, avoiding a task or situation, getting attention, calming themselves down, or as a response to pain or discomfort. Problem behaviour can have more than one function for a child and can trigger strong emotions from others which may make it difficult to think about the behaviour dispassionately and to describe it objectively.

> John screamed to get attention from Sue. With support from the early intervention therapist, Sue worked on ignoring the screaming so that it was no longer functional for John. The early intervention therapist also helped Sue and Mike teach John an alternative appropriate behaviour to fulfil the same function, in this case initially teaching John to go to Sue and touch her arm. Later he learnt to show her a picture of what he wanted. In this way John learnt how to get attention without screaming. Behaviours may have more than one function for a child. For example, John also had great difficulty coping with noisy crowded environments and would also start to scream in shopping malls, having learnt that in this situation screaming usually resulted in Sue making a hasty exit. In this situation ignoring the behaviour was not an option for Sue plus it was unlikely to be effective, as ignoring the behaviour won't make the noisy, confusing environment (A–Antecedent) go away. Sue and John's early intervention therapist worked on introducing John to noisy, crowded environments gradually for brief periods and making the experience as positive as possible for him. Sue avoided taking him with her when she needed to do the big family grocery shop.

It is likely there is more than one behaviour you want to change, but realistically you can focus only on one thing at a time. You will find that successfully managing one problem behaviour will have a positive ripple effect on other behaviours and other aspects of life for you and your child. When thinking about behaviour change we tend to focus on consequences, especially negative ones such as punishment. Punishment frequently doesn't work for children with autism for a variety of reasons; for example, they may enjoy the time alone in 'time out'.

> Being taken out to the car park at the shopping mall and making him sit in the car was exactly what John wanted and actually reinforced his screaming.

For any strategy to be effective, you first have to understand the cause (or trigger) of the behaviour which will help you look for ways to stop the behaviour happening. For example, many children with autism are very sensitive to some types of light touch and don't like the labels on the back of their clothes touching their skin. It is simplest to remove the labels and prevent the sensation that triggers the behaviour. If the cause of the behaviour is an attempt to communicate then it is important to teach alternative behaviours so that the function of the behaviour is still achieved, otherwise it is possible that your child will come up with another, possibly worse, unwanted behaviour to achieve the same function.

> If Sue had tried to stop John screaming to get her attention without teaching him an appropriate way to do this he may have started hitting her or hitting himself instead.

When developing a wanted behaviour, make sure that what you want your child to learn is reasonable based upon their abilities. It may be necessary to break down the learning task into smaller steps and consider what prompts your child may need to succeed. You can gradually reduce the prompts as they learn. The way you communicate is crucial. Work out the most effective way to communicate with your child, as described earlier in this chapter. This will usually involve showing as well as telling them what you want them to do. Modelling the behaviour may also help (more on this below). Be aware that when you first put a strategy in place to manage behaviour there may be an initial increase in the unwanted behaviour as your child tries harder to use a strategy that has worked for them in the past.

> Jane's behaviour when she started preschool could have benefited from an A–B–C approach. The function of Jane's difficult behaviour when leaving home and arriving at preschool was clearly protest. The first step would be to determine what it was about the preschool situation that was difficult for her: was it lack of predictability and structure, in which case a visual schedule at home and at preschool could be used to help her understand what was going to happen; or was it the noise and activity of the other children, in which case could she come at a quieter time or use a different entrance or have her own special quiet place at preschool to go to. Alternatively, she could have been distressed at being left by Louise (which would be evident in other settings as well), in which case a visual schedule showing Jane the program for the day and when it was home time with a photo of Louise might be enough to reassure her. Can Louise and the staff make preschool a rewarding and positive experience for Jane? These are all potential strategies to be explored. If the behaviour has more than one trigger or function for Jane, then more than one strategy may be required.

You may also recognise that in some situations you have been provoked to give a negative reaction. For example, sometimes children with autism find the changes in another person's face and voice when they are angry or sad interesting and will provoke that behaviour without understanding the effect they are having on another person's feelings. If you know this is happening you can make a plan to prevent it happening again. You can either change your own behaviour (don't react), or work towards changing your child's behaviour (teach them how to interact with you positively).

Consistency is important, so you need to make sure things are being done the same way in different settings, like at home, child care and granny's house. If you and all your child's carers can agree on consistent ways to respond, you'll effect positive change sooner. You need to be sure there are no weak links in the chain.

We all love rewards. Sometimes a change in behaviour will bring about automatic rewards but additional planned rewards can assist during the early stages.

If you've given it enough time and done everything by the book and the behaviour hasn't changed it is time to go back to the drawing board. It helps to have some team support and it is necessary to be patient and flexible. As much as is possible, put yourself in your child's shoes and think again about what the function of the behaviour is for your child. What is triggering it and what is maintaining it? Can you and your child communicate about it? Is the alternative you are trying to teach achievable and rewarding enough? Are you teaching an alternative skill using small enough steps and the right prompts for your child? Not all behaviours are changed on the first attempt.

If the behaviour is changing in the right direction there is likely to be a general positive effect and fewer problem behaviours as a result. For a summary of the key behaviour management principles that can be used in a variety of different settings, see Table 2 overleaf.

We'll provide further examples of how these can be applied to different situations and at different ages throughout the following chapters.

Table 2: Principles and practices for reducing unwanted behaviours and achieving wanted behaviours

Key steps	Strategies
Prioritise	Choose the behaviour having the biggest impact on your child, your family and others.
Describe exactly the behaviour	Write down exactly what happens when, where, with whom and how often. Focus on what you can observe, not what you think people are feeling or thinking.
Work out the trigger and the consequences: A–B–C	Focus on what you think is triggering the behaviour (the antecedent) and then what is maintaining it (the consequence).
Work out the function of the behaviour	The function of the behaviour may not be immediately obvious and you may have to test out several theories. Always check for a physical cause for the problem behaviour first.
Develop a strategy	Aim to prevent the behaviour by changing the environment, teaching the child an alternative way to respond, or a combination of strategies. Think of the consequence, which could be maintaining the behaviour, and look at ways to change that. Keep in mind the overall function of the behaviour and ensure that your child has another appropriate way of achieving that function.
Teach an alternative wanted behaviour	Be very clear about what it is you want your child to learn. Give your child the support (prompts) they need to succeed and gradually reduce the prompts as they learn. This is called errorless learning.
Make sure everyone knows the procedure and it is done consistently	It is essential that everyone around the child is consistent and responds to the problem behaviour in the same way and works on teaching the same replacement behaviour the same way.

Key steps	Strategies
Reward the child for appropriate behaviour — ensure it works for them	A fundamental principle of behaviour and learning is that we repeat behaviours that reward us. Behaviour management will be most effective when unwanted behaviours are replaced by wanted behaviours that your child finds equally or more rewarding.
Evaluate the strategy	Keep a record of the times and places the unwanted behaviour occurs. There may be an initial increase but then, if the strategy is working, you will see a reduction in the behaviour over time.
Maintain the strategy	Maintain the strategy until the behaviour is established (for a wanted behaviour) or no longer present (for an unwanted behaviour). Remember that if the triggers and the consequences return, the behaviour is likely to come back.
Consider generalisation	Your child may have difficulty generalising something they have learnt in one setting or context to other settings or contexts. You may need to teach the wanted behaviour in different contexts (times, places, people).
If the behaviour is still a problem	Review your theory about the function, the trigger and the consequence of the behaviour. Have you successfully taught an alternative way to achieve the same function? Is the new behaviour equally rewarding? Is everyone around your child being consistent?
Work as a team	Work with others to ensure consistency and to get the support *you* need. Other people might observe things you may have missed.
Managing change	Plan for change. Collect information about what is going to happen, when, where and with whom. Prepare your child for the change by explaining what is going to happen in a way they can understand.

EARLY INTERVENTIONS

The evidence we have tells us that the most effective interventions for young children with autism are those based on learning, which we will discuss further below. There are many other interventions for autism that are not based on learning that may be suggested or promoted. The toddler and preschool years are when you will be offered early intervention. You are likely to be exploring all possible interventions in the hope that starting early will bring the greatest benefit to your child.

Interventions can differ in what they target. Some aim to change the core characteristics required for a diagnosis of autism (deficits in social communication and restricted, repetitive behaviours), while others target characteristics that are associated with autism (inattention, hyperactivity and anxiety). The delivery of each intervention can be different. Some are ingested interventions, like prescribed medications or nutritional therapies, while others involve exposure to different environments, like animal therapies. Some interventions are called 'complementary' or 'alternative' medicine, which are general terms for therapies that are not part of conventional practice, used either as an alternative to or alongside mainstream care. Some come from non-western cultures and others are established for some specific problems, like taking vitamin B6 for vitamin B6 deficiency, but are considered complementary or alternative for others, like giving vitamin B6 for autism. Once there is evidence that a complementary or alternative medicine is effective it loses that label.

It is worth noting that no medication has been demonstrated to change the core characteristics of autism. Some prescribed medications have been shown to be effective in minimising behaviours that are unwanted or impede learning, such as hyperactivity, impulsivity, aggression, anxiety, self-injurious and obsessive/compulsive behaviours (see sections in chapters 7 and 9 for further discussion). No complementary and alternative therapies have been demonstrated to change the core characteristics of autism. Some complementary or alternative approaches are also discussed in relation to specific problems in later chapters (see also Resources at the end of this chapter).

There is no shortage of available interventions for autism, but if they are not known to be effective, then you need to be cautious because the possibility of causing harm could be greater than the potential benefit. You should consider whether the intervention could cause distress and financial hardship for your family and whether doing the intervention prevents you from taking up one that is known to be beneficial. One parent put it this way: 'One of the things I have found difficult to deal with is that so many well-meaning people have their pet theories on what will "cure" or help your ASD child. Of course they are only trying to offer you something that might help, and it is nice to receive support and advice, as opposed to straight-out criticism. But as a parent you feel obliged to investigate and evaluate every option ... Investigating all these things can totally wear you out. It takes so much time and energy, not to mention money!'[1]

LEARNING-BASED INTERVENTIONS

Learning-based interventions may be behavioural or developmental in focus, and they can use different methods or target different behaviours. Some are defined by the training of the professionals who offer them, like speech therapists; some focus on one characteristic or area of skill development, such as the Picture Exchange Communication System (PECS) which targets communication. Others, such as Pivotal Response Training (PRT), the Early Start Denver Model (ESDM) and the TEACCH® program, use a variety of methods and focus on a broad range of behaviour, development and learning (see the Glossary for more information about these interventions). There are also many unnamed early intervention programs, often known only by the name of the organisation or service that provides them, that use a variety of methods and that have a broad focus that are suitable for children with autism. By using more than one intervention approach, it is possible to address the many needs of your child with autism as they arise and change. Although many therapies are called 'early intervention', they can also be used beyond the preschool years (see Resources at the end of this chapter).

There are so many suggested forms of early intervention for autism that parents often talk about the maze they navigate trying to find the 'right' one for their child's age and stage. This is especially the case at the beginning of the process when you have just found out that your child has, or is suspected to have, autism. The internet is a mixed blessing with a vast amount of information and a range of claims and counterclaims, often highly emotional, about how effective different interventions are. In Chapter 10 we provide some information about how to filter some of this information. Personal endorsements, anecdotal information and testimonials are very common and very hard to ignore when you read or hear that an intervention has 'cured' a child. Of course, as a parent, you want the best for your child.

A step-wise approach is a good way to navigate the maze. The first step is to understand the different types of interventions that may be available and the second step is knowing where to find reliable information about how effective these interventions have been for children with autism. The third step is to find out if the intervention you have chosen is available, affordable and adds value to the other interventions your child is accessing. The final step is making sure a treatment or intervention your child is receiving is achieving the goals you have set and is not causing adverse effects. In this chapter we are going to provide information for step one. We provide information for step two throughout Chapter 10.

TYPES OF LEARNING-BASED INTERVENTIONS

Learning-based interventions come from our understanding of communication, behaviour change, and learning. They are designed to help your child learn a new behaviour or skill or unlearn an unwanted behaviour.

The first recognised learning-based intervention in autism was applied behavioural analysis, usually known as ABA, which was developed in the 1960s. ABA programs at that time were prescriptive and focused on teaching appropriate behaviour by breaking down complex tasks into smaller, more achievable steps and rewarding the child for a correct response (a novel idea at the time). A skill was taught in a series of small steps called discrete trials (stimulus–response–reinforcement) which were repeated many times. For example, a child would be taught to say a word by providing the stimulus 'say cat' and the response 'cat' would be rewarded with a star sticker. Prior to the first use of ABA, children with autism were usually considered uneducable and institutionalisation was recommended. Today, ABA programs can be described as traditional/Lovaas programs or contemporary ABA. Traditional ABA adheres to the original approach of using discrete trials repeatedly (also called 'massed practice') and the program is delivered intensively for 20–40 hours a week. These programs are sometimes also called 'early intensive behavioural intervention' (EIBI). Contemporary ABA programs, such as Pivotal Response Training (PRT), incorporate what has been learnt about child development and social communication development in recent decades and focus more on learning in everyday settings using naturally occuring reinforcement.

New understandings about child development have given us a better understanding of the way early social communication skills develop, which has led to interventions that focus on social communication and building positive relationships (engagement). These programs, for example DIRFloortime®, focus on initiation and spontaneity in communication by following a child's interests and motivations, building on a child's communicative repertoire, even if this is unconventional, and using more natural activities and events to support the development of communication.

Today, learning-based programs increasingly combine behavioural and developmental approaches to autism. They are also likely to incorporate approaches to managing the environment, use of visually-based information to compensate for auditory processing problems, as well as directly teaching your child. These interventions can vary widely in intensity and treatment philosophy and may target a specific area of development or set goals across all areas of functioning. Learning-based programs may occur in the home, a clinic or centre, or within another setting, like child care or school. Effective programs will be taught across the home, school and community to ensure the skills your child is learning are functional and able to be applied in more than one setting or context (see Resources at the end of this chapter).

YOUR ROLE IN EARLY INTERVENTION

As a parent, you play a critical role in supporting your child's learning and your involvement is a key ingredient to the success of any early intervention program. It is important that you form a good working relationship with the professionals working with your child, and to do this you will need a clear idea of both your and their expectations and a willingness to work together. To work effectively on a program with your professionals you will need to acknowledge that their many roles may mean you need to schedule meetings or negotiate when and how you will communicate. You won't like every professional you meet, but that doesn't mean you won't be able to form a relationship with them that is in the best interests of your child. You will need to trust their professional knowledge and experience and you should expect that they show this in the way they interact with you and your child. They should also value your understanding of your child.

Important characteristics you might look for in the professionals you work with are:
- The ability to listen.
- The ability to explain things in a way that you understand. If you don't understand it is fine to ask for a further explanation.
- Being well informed about autism and the range of interventions available, as well as being able to recommend useful resources.

- The ability to acknowledge when they can't address something either because of time constraints or because it is outside their expertise. Both of these situations could arise and should not diminish that professional in your eyes, as long as they discuss how they will work towards resolving the issue you have raised.
- A willingness to help you assess evidence and make the best decisions for your child and then assist in monitoring outcomes once interventions have been decided.

If you feel you do not have a good working relationship with a professional providing early intervention for your child, make a time with them to discuss what you think is needed. It can be helpful to first make sure others think there is sufficient reason for concern. If it is possible that your wellbeing or a high level of stress is influencing your thoughts and actions, then think first about looking after yourself (see Chapter 4). As described in Chapter 3, if you don't think you are able to have that conversation alone, then seek help from family or friends.

If, despite your best efforts, you are still unable to establish a good working relationship, it is reasonable to ask if it is possible for another early intervention professional to become involved. Professionals working in teams may have the flexibility to offer another person within that team, or alternatively may be able to recommend another service that could meet your child's needs.

In an increasing number of early intervention programs, parents are also being given a primary role in delivering the intervention. These are known as parent-mediated interventions. In particular, there has been a recent rapid growth of interventions based on parent training for toddler-aged children with autism in North America and the UK as a result of earlier identification, desire to provide intervention as soon as possible, and a need to work within available resources. Interventions being delivered by parents are as varied those delivered by professionals described above. Examples range from home-based, parent-delivered intensive behavioural programs (such as EIBI) to the Hanen Program® called More Than Words® (MTW).

The same principles apply to choosing a parent-mediated intervention as for those where the professional works directly with your child. Your choice will depend on what is likely to fit your goals and priorities, based on your child's strengths and needs and to some extent on your personal style and preference. Cost is also likely to be a consideration. You may choose a combination. The evidence for the effectiveness of parent-mediated intervention is best in the area of language development, both in expression and comprehension, with good outcomes in parent–child synchrony for sharing attention and interactions. There is also some evidence to suggest a reduction in the severity of autism characteristics.

There are many reasons why you may decide not to undertake a parent-mediated early intervention program with your child, especially a highly intensive one. Before embarking on this type of program think about whether you have the time, whether you want to separate your role as a parent from your role as your child's therapist, and whether this approach is best for your emotional and physical wellbeing (see Resources at the end of this chapter).

EVIDENCE FOR EARLY INTERVENTION

The evidence for learning-based early interventions for autism is now summarised in many systematic reviews and summaries. More than twenty learning-based interventions have been found to have some evidence for effectiveness in preschoolers, but with consistent findings that these programs help some but not all children with autism. Much of the research evaluating interventions has been done in settings where the quality of the intervention can be tightly controlled, however this is much more difficult to do outside research studies. There are also gaps in the evidence available about how different types of interventions compare or add value to one another. As a result, we often don't have the sort of evidence we need to make 'real-world' decisions about what is best. Gaps also exist in our understanding about how to predict which children are most likely to benefit from which intervention, at which stage in development different interventions are most effective, and what the right amount of intervention is to achieve best outcomes. Current research is trying to fill those gaps (see Resources at the end of this chapter).

We do know that programs that work for children with autism share many of the key features in Table 3. Good programs address the core issues of autism, such as social communication, and also take into account related problems like anxiety, hyperactivity and poor concentration. Good programs teach skills in a highly supportive environment and work towards having children participate in more complex, natural environments with a wider range of people. Autism is a condition that straddles the domains of many different professions in terms of its definition, diagnosis, education and care. Professionals need to work with other professionals from different disciplines, and the development and implementation of intervention strategies must include parents, teachers, peers and the person with autism.

> John started an early intervention program when he was three. The best available option for John was a home-based early intervention service, which John started after a six-month wait when he was three-and-a-half. John had home-based early intervention for eighteen months. An early intervention therapist came to visit John and Sue at home to assess John and develop a program. She came once a fortnight and worked with them on John's program, adjusting it as he met the goals and new priorities came up. Sue worked on the program with John every day and tried to incorporate the program into the family's daily routines, especially bath time and mealtimes to help John learn to use new skills across different situations. After twelve months, when John was just four-and-a-half, the therapist started a gradual program to introduce John to a local preschool.

Amidst the debate about the relative merits of the different programs and the theories that underpin them, John's parents found a program that worked for him and for them and that assisted with his transition to preschool and school.

Table 3: Key features of programs that work

Key feature	Important elements
Provide program content for children with autism	Develop the child's ability to: attend to elements of the environment; imitate others; comprehend and use language or alternative communication; play appropriately with toys; engage socially with others; manage change and transition; and recognise and regulate their own and others' emotions.
Highly supportive learning environment	Appropriate environmental supports, structured teaching, and visual supports set up in the child's environment to assist with learning and making sense of their world.
Predictability and routine	Routines are established within and between sessions, which are supported visually where appropriate and extend into family life and other settings. Learning to manage changes in routine should also be incorporated.
A functional approach to challenging behaviours	Prevent unwanted behaviours by increasing interest and motivation, structuring the environment, and positive behaviour support including teaching alternative appropriate skills, and communication strategies to replace unwanted behaviours. If unwanted behaviours persist, use the approaches described in Table 2 (see page 84).
Inclusion and peer support	Include typically developing peers when and where possible, in a supported program.
Encourage independence	Promote independent functioning throughout the intervention program.

Key feature	Important elements
Outcome-focused	Be clear what expected outcomes are and monitor to assess progress towards these goals.
Transition support	A focus on coping with change and transition. Integration between the program and the next stage for the child and preparation for change, whether it is major (transition to school or to another therapeutic setting) or minor (a change in the route to preschool).
Family involvement	Families involved in assessment and in program development and implementation. Families supported to use strategies taught as part of the interventions at home, and to encourage communication, social interaction and effective behaviour management at home and in the community. Parent groups, sibling groups and other types of emotional support available to assist with stresses encountered by families of children with autism. Provision of good information to families about autism and about services.
Use of visual supports	Development of methods to allow expressive and receptive communication, and visually cued instruction and visual information to provide the child with a predictable and readily understood environment.
Multidisciplinary collaborative approach	Assessments and programs provided by a number professionals, including speech therapists, psychologists and teachers. Professionals work either as part of a geographically co-located team or in separate locations but in close communication with each other. Collaboration and teamwork extend to the child care or educational setting.
Focus on motivation and creative use of special interests	Incorporate management of preoccupations and rituals into programs and focus on strengths and special interests to engage the child in learning to provide naturally occurring reinforcement.

While there are still some learning-based programs which adhere to one theory, either behavioural or developmental, interventions and programs for young children with autism increasingly use multiple approaches and are more similar than they are different. Many programs do not have a specific name, other than the name of the organisation or service that provides them, which makes it difficult to work out what approach they are based on.

It is likely your child will need a combination of different approaches based on their age and stage of development and on what they need to learn and that the approaches needed will change over time. Whatever program you are considering for your child there are key questions you can ask, as shown in the box below.

QUESTIONS TO ASK WHEN CONSIDERING AN INTERVENTION FOR YOUR CHILD[2]

» What are the specific aims of the program?

» Are there any medical or physical risks?

» What assessments of individual children are carried out prior to the intervention?

» What is the evidence base for this intervention?

» What evaluation methods have been used to assess the outcome of the intervention?

» Do the proponents of the treatment program have a financial stake in its adoption?

» What is known about the long-term effects of this treatment?

» How much does it cost?

» How much time will be involved?

RESOURCES

General information about development and behaviour during the toddler and preschool years

> http://raisingchildren.net.au/toddlers/toddlers.html

> http://raisingchildren.net.au/preschoolers/preschoolers.html

Communication skill assessment using The Pragmatics Profile of Everyday Communication Skills in Children

> wwwedit.wmin.ac.uk/psychology/pp/children.htm

Positive behaviour support guide (developed for school-aged children but applicable to younger children)

> www.autismtraining.com.au/public/index.cfm?action=showPublicContent&assetCategoryId=1143

A–B–C approaches to behaviour management and recording sheets

> www.amaze.org.au/uploads/2011/08/Fact-Sheet-Behaviour-Management-Strategies-Aug-2011.pdf

> www.iidc.indiana.edu/?pageId=444

Information about managing behaviour

> www.autismspeaks.org/sites/default/files/section_5.pdf

> www.autism.org.uk/living-with-autism/understanding-behaviour/challenging-behaviour/challenging-behaviour-in-children-with-an-asd.aspx

> www.autismtraining.com.au/public/index.cfm?action=showPublicContent&assetCategoryId=1029

Definitions and information about complementary or alternative approaches

> http://nccam.nih.gov/health/whatiscam

> www.compmed.umm.edu/cochrane_about.asp

Early intervention reviews

> http://autismpdc.fpg.unc.edu/sites/autismpdc.fpg.unc.edu/files/2014-EBP-Report.pdf

> www.dss.gov.au/our-responsibilities/disability-and-carers/program-services/for-people-with-disability/helping-children-with-autism

> http://effectivehealthcare.ahrq.gov/index.cfm/search-for-guides-reviews-and-reports/?productid=1945&pageaction=displayproduct

Early intensive behavioural intervention systematic review

http://onlinelibrary.wiley.com/doi/10.1002/14651858.CD009260.pub2/abstract

Parent-mediated interventions systematic review

http://onlinelibrary.wiley.com/doi/10.1002/14651858.CD009774.pub2/abstract

Summaries for some interventions

http://raisingchildren.net.au/articles/therapies_guide_faqs.html

Guidelines for good practice in autism early intervention

www.dss.gov.au/sites/default/files/documents/11_2012/early_intervention_practice_guidlines.pdf

The roles of different professionals in autism

www.therapyconnect.amaze.org.au/

CHAPTER 6

PROBLEMS IN THE PRESCHOOL YEARS

Many of the problems described below are not specific to autism. They may occur in any child but in autism the cause of the behaviour and its severity or intensity might be different. It is also possible that it may take longer to change a behaviour or address a problem because your child with autism may have different communication needs, is not motivated by social interaction, or has a different range of abilities. The reasons for an unwanted behaviour in children with autism may also be harder to identify and more complex.

SLEEP

Sleeping problems are common for both children with autism and typically developing children. On average a toddler needs ten to twelve hours of sleep a night and may benefit from an additional one to two hours during the day as well. A preschooler needs eleven to thirteen hours per night, but will sleep less during the day or not at all. Different people have varying sleep patterns and sleep requirements, but if your child is sleeping less than this you should not simply assume they have a minimal sleep requirement. Your child will always need more sleep than you (see Resources at the end of this chapter).

Most sleep problems are due to unwanted behaviours that affect sleeping patterns. If a child has only ever gone to sleep with the television on or with a certain person with them, then they may be unable to fall asleep without this association. Some children become anxious on getting in to bed, either thinking about the events of the day or worrying about something associated with the night, like the dark. Other children get into the habit of going to bed late and waking up late. This can happen because parents have not created limits around bedtime. Others get up and play in the middle of the night.

Children with autism can have more than one sleep problem. The behaviours that are associated with waking can be more disruptive than for children who don't have autism because of a lack of concern about disturbing others, and they can be more resistant to usual behavioural strategies. You may find that your child needs even more sleep-related structure and direction because they do not pick up on cues around bedtime, which are often linked to social cues. They may have particular problems or behaviours that make bedtime more challenging (like being unwilling to part with an object of special interest or being more anxious in the dark), and they may also react against behavioural management more strongly and more persistently. It is also likely that your child will have more than one unwanted behaviour that you would like to change.

> Jane had substantial sleep problems that her parents found hard to manage before she was diagnosed as having autism. The problems Jane had are not un-common, including resistance to going to bed and a pattern of being put to bed after falling asleep, but then waking and being distressed.

For children, sleep is even more important than for adults, so resolving sleep issues should be high on your list of priorities. Adequate sleep is a fundamental requirement for physical, emotional and social wellbeing. There is no direct link between limited sleep and problems with growth, except at the extremes of sleep deprivation, but the body does require sleep to function and grow optimally. Children also find it hard to attend and learn if they have had insufficient sleep, while as adults we know that a lack of sleep changes the way we react physically, socially and emotionally. If you and your child get enough sleep on any one night you're going to have a different day than the one you would have without enough sleep. Over time, sufficient sleep will lead to an accumulation of positive benefits, including improved engagement and learning.

SLEEP PROBLEMS THAT ARE NOT BEHAVIOURAL

Your child may experience some sleep problems that are not behavioural. On rare occasions, a child's sleep will appear to be interrupted by night terrors. A child experiencing night terrors will usually be sitting up screaming but will not, in fact, be awake. The simplest evidence-based intervention for night terrors is to wake your child every night for a week just prior to the time the night terror has been occurring, say within the preceding hour. This usually helps break the cycle.

Nightmares also can disrupt sleep, but are usually short-lived. Soothing your child's distress and offering pleasant distractions is usually the best course. If they have enough understanding of language you can reassure them that dreams don't come true and tell them pleasant things they can think about instead.

Is there a biological reason why your child isn't sleeping? There are very few biological reasons why children don't sleep, but there are some important biological reasons why your child's sleep could be disturbed. If your child is snoring every night and they have episodes where it looks and sounds as though they have stopped breathing before the snoring returns, you should consult your doctor. This could be obstructive sleep apnoea and, although they remain asleep, their quality of sleep will be poor and they won't be rested in the morning. If your child wakes repeatedly and seems to be in pain, it is also important to seek medical advice. Similarly, if your child wakes thirsty, needs to drink and is weeing throughout the night a medical assessment is needed. These problems are not specific to children with autism but they may be harder to identify. These behaviours usually follow a pattern where the child goes off to sleep, but then experiences the problems while asleep or wakes because of them.

BEHAVIOURAL APPROACHES FOR SLEEP ISSUES

How can you increase wanted sleep behaviours or minimise unwanted behaviours that interfere with sleep? Bedtime is a time when routines and even rituals can be very helpful. Bedtime routines and good habits are also known as 'sleep hygiene'. Habits that can be helpful are having a set bedtime, having a set place to sleep with some objects that your child finds soothing or reassuring, having a few things that are always associated with going to sleep (like a glass of milk and a bedtime story), and being away from too much noise. If a child is anxious then relaxation techniques and strategies to 'put away worries' can be very helpful. Some things interfere with developing good sleep behaviour. Televisions, tablets and computers are all mentally stimulating and should be turned off in bedrooms at night, and removed if possible. Visual technology should never be part of a bedtime routine, except as part of a planned sleep improvement strategy with a staged withdrawal.

Although there is little evidence about interventions to improve sleep in children with autism, there is every reason to expect that the same approaches used for typically developing children or those with other developmental problems like attention deficit hyperactivity disorder (ADHD) will be effective. Weighted blankets have been shown not to work in one randomised controlled trial (see Resources at the end of this chapter).

Jane had problems both getting off to sleep and waking in the night. Establishing a positive bedtime routine and bringing Jane's bedtime gradually toward the desired time would be the first steps to take. Jane's night-waking and screaming were not night terrors or nightmares; they were due to her distress at waking in a situation she was not expecting to be in, because she was in a location she had resisted falling asleep in and was not in the same place that she fell asleep. Once Jane is settling to sleep in the place she will stay overnight, it is likely that the night-waking and screaming will also resolve. These behavioural techniques use the 'managing change' approaches to encourage wanted behaviours and reduce unwanted ones described in Table 2.

Behavioural sleep interventions can take a lot of effort. They are especially difficult because they take place at the end of the day when everyone is tired and they can be wearying for others, especially siblings if they share a room. This is not the sort of endeavour to embark on half-heartedly and consistency is vital amongst all carers and parents. We recommend professional input and support along the way to both develop a plan that is most likely to succeed for your child, you and your family and also to provide you with support and 'troubleshooting' advice.

MEDICATION AS A 'CYCLE BREAKER'

Sometimes you may not get to step one of a behavioural intervention. This is the time that medication may be helpful. In this situation medication is being used to either reduce a problem that is preventing a bedtime routine being established or to offer a behaviour 'cycle breaker' by inducing sleep and creating one step of the wanted behaviour. If, for example, your child is afraid of being in their room on their own, then a suitable medication may reduce their anxiety or may provide an opportunity for some positive experiences that allow them to build on that success. Medication should only be used under supervision from your doctor and should only be one part of the approach toward improving sleep behaviours. Medical supervision is needed for the prescription of appropriate drugs and also to monitor possible side effects. With your doctor you should plan the outcomes you want and how to record them. By reducing a problem, medication can assist a stepwise approach toward wanted sleep behaviours. Once these are established, then it is time to wean your child off the medication, again under medical supervision. Some agents can cause serious health problems if they are stopped suddenly. A decision about the possible value of a medication for improving sleep needs to take into account the potential risks and benefits as well as an assessment of whether the desired goal has been achieved.

There are many different types of medication that can be used to help sleep including melatonin, a hormone known to assist with sleep onset and to play a key role in the natural sleep cycle. Melatonin does not prolong sleep duration and earlier onset of sleep may mean earlier wakening, which might not be a benefit for you. Clonidine is known to be effective as a treatment for ADHD and can also improve night-time settling. Other medications that are sedating agents include chloral hydrate and antihistamines, like promethazine and trimeprazine. Some children have a paradoxical response to antihistamines and become more active, so they are not right for everyone. Antipsychotic medication and antidepressants can also be used for sleep problems but should only be prescribed for toddlers and preschool children under very specific circumstances, like severe anxiety or for a severe repetitive behaviour that is disrupting sleep. Each of these medications has different risks and benefits that your doctor will be able to discuss with you. As well as monitoring wanted sleep behaviours, side effects should also be monitored.

WHEN NOTHING YOU'VE TRIED HAS WORKED

If nothing has helped then don't give up. Go back to the professionals you know or seek advice about others who may be able to assist. Let them know what you have tried and the barriers to success. By writing down everything you have done so far, it may help to work out things that haven't been tried or strategies that might be more effective. You should also think about the things that must be achieved to ensure your child's safety and your ability to get some sleep, including the use of other services and modifications to your home, if necessary. You and your child's sleep is a priority.

MANAGING CHANGE

Change is an inevitable part of life. Change and unpredictability are frequently very difficult for children with autism who may go to extreme lengths to maintain routine and sameness in their lives. General pointers about managing behaviours and identifying the trigger are described in Chapter 5. Because change is a common trigger for unwanted behaviours, we have provided a couple of different approaches here that could work for you and your child as well.

The first way to address an unwanted behaviour, like a tantrum, that is due to change is to prevent change occurring by managing the child's environment. If a change of route home from preschool was triggering tantrums, it may be reasonable to take the same route to and from school every day. This is quite usual for many children. However, there may be times when there are changes that can't be predicted or prevented, like roadworks on the usual route to preschool and you have to go a different way. So while we are reducing problem behaviours by managing triggers and maintaining routines, it is also important to improve your child's ability to cope with change.

A common approach is to introduce change in very small increments so your child can get used to it gradually. This will require careful preparation. Breaking down change into small steps is not always easy for adults and you may benefit from professional input. The sorts of changes you might make as a first step would include stopping at a different place on the same route, changing sides of who walks near the road but on the same route, or changing the role of who decides when it is time to cross the road. You could also provide some commentary about what you are planning and doing as you go. For example, you might stop on the way and say, 'Look! A big tree'. Anxiety, distress or unwanted behaviour created by small changes will be less severe and intense than the response to a major change. Think about how you can communicate visually as well as verbally with your child about change. In this example you might have drawings or photos showing the route to preschool, or you could show your child a variation to the route you are planning on a map. You might also take a picture of the tree and add it to the route, and talk about it later in the day using the drawings and photos. Remember, keep your language simple, clear, concrete and brief. Being able to communicate with your child is a key part of this process and the use of visual supports, such as schedules, is very effective in helping children with autism learn to manage change and to trust others.

> Siew's parents found the visual aids his speech therapist had given them a great asset for managing change. Without his schedule Siew found change very difficult to understand and deal with and became very distressed. When something different happened Hong Yuan noticed that Siew seemed to understand a lot less than at other times. She found it very helpful to show him what was planned as well as to tell him.

Sometimes we don't even realise that what we are planning will be a big change. After the event it is easy to look at any situation in which there have been difficulties and realise how things could have been done differently, for example Todd's birthday party.

> Jessica had a birthday party for Todd when he turned four. She invited a small group of children from his preschool as well as his cousins. Todd found the experience very stressful, refused to join in any of the games or eat any party food, ripped the paper off his presents without acknowledgement, despite prompting

from his mother, and showed little interest in the contents. Finally he shut himself in his room, refusing to come out until everyone had left.

For many children with autism, birthday parties represent their worst nightmare — lots of noise, crowding, loud or unexpected noises, strange food and unpredictable behaviour.

With hindsight the party for Todd may have worked better with more planning and opportunities for Todd to understand all the different aspects of the party and expected behaviours. Also with the benefit of hindsight, it is evident that a party with lots of people, presents and games is unlikely to be a success if less complex social interactions have been difficult.

RESTRICTED AND REPETITIVE BEHAVIOURS

Restricted and repetitive behaviours are a key feature of autism and can be very different from child to child. Some are particular movements, also described in Chapter 8 in the section on stereotypies. Others are vocal, visual or involve other senses. It can be difficult to identify the triggers or function for some restricted and repetitive behaviours. Varied triggers include seeking pleasurable sensory stimulation or attempts to reduce sensory input, attempts to block out other events or environmental factors that are not understood or stressful, or a deep interest in an object. If the triggered behaviour serves a desired function then it will be more resistant to change. The approach to managing restricted and repetitive behaviours follows the broad principles described in Chapter 5. Of note, a restricted or repetitive behaviour may be your child's way of managing their stress — a coping strategy for some unavoidable situations. If repetitive behaviours are a response to a stressful situation and a way for your child to cope with it, you must think carefully about how much of a priority it is to change that behaviour and recognise that you need to reduce the stress triggering it or teach your child an alternative way to manage stress. This may be necessary if the repetitive or restricted behaviour is having a negative effect on their social opportunities, and this will need to be considered amongst the other risks and benefits of behaviour change.

SENSORY PROBLEMS

Sensory problems are common during the preschool years and can include becoming upset at some sounds (loud hand dryers in public toilets) and some visual stimuli (dressed-up characters), and also avoidance of some activities involving touch (messy play, hair washing) or seeking out some sensations, like being soothed by touching a certain type of fabric. More unusual behaviours that indicate sensory problems include indifference to pain, excessive smelling of objects and long periods of staring at flickering or certain patterns of light. These are seen in autism and also with specific problems like not being able to see or hear. Your child with autism is likely to have a more extreme and inconsolable reaction to a sensory stimulus that they find unpleasant and also likely to have sensory-seeking behaviours that are more persistent and difficult to change. These behaviours have been noted since the original description of autism and are now included as one possible diagnostic criteria (see Chapter 3). Some professionals call this a 'sensory processing disorder'.

Sensory issues and problems can have a major impact on your child's ability to attend, respond and learn so the effective management of sensory issues in autism is potentially of great benefit. Environmental management can be effective and the approaches you can use are similar to those you have read about for other behaviour problems (see Chapter 5) and that come up again as useful strategies during the school years (see chapters 7 and 9). If possible, plan ahead and either avoid the sensory stimuli that upsets your child or visit at a time when it is likely noise or other sensations they dislike will be less. If the latter approach is possible, like going to the pool at a time when fewer people are there, and it is successful, then you may be able to very gradually move toward times when there are more people at the pool. You should also warn your child before going to a place where sensations they find unpleasant will occur. For example, you could warn them, using verbal or visual information, that there is a possibility there will be loud sounds where you are going. Plan with your child what you will both do if there are loud sounds. You might show them that they can wear ear muffs or ear plugs, if they tolerate these, and also that it is all right to let you know when they would like to leave. If the unpleasant stimulus occurs at a place your child attends frequently, like child care, discuss the problem with other people involved and plan a quiet place for your child. If you are worried that the problem could occur at an event your child has been invited to, like a party, discuss the problem, how to prevent it and what to do if it occurs with the people involved. Being forewarned and having a good plan may prevent the problem and will minimise the impact of it if it can't be avoided.

If problems persist, occupational therapists are trained to provide interventions to manage your child's sensory issues and will have other environmental management techniques they can recommend, or they will decide if it is best to teach your child to manage their sensory issues via desensitisation approaches.

Two other types of therapy for sensory issues have received considerable attention, and are usually referred to as 'auditory integration training' (AIT) and 'sensory integration therapy'. These therapies are based on the theory that the use of sound and movement and other sensory inputs leads to improved processing of that one sensory mode (e.g. sounds or touch) and may lead to improvements in other brain functions that enhance learning. For example, sound therapies are designed to reduce sound sensitivities and, as a result, improve sound processing abilities. Some sound therapies claim to improve all areas of development and functioning. There is no evidence that sound therapies are effective in changing auditory sensitivities or behaviour. Some sound therapies have not been investigated thoroughly while others have not shown positive results, like auditory integration therapy (see Resources at the end of this chapter).

Todd had auditory integration training (AIT) when he was four which Jessica felt improved his behaviour for a while, although his father Joseph disagreed.

Other sensory integration therapies provide vestibular (balance), tactile (touch), and/or proprioceptive (sense of where the body is in space) stimulation. Activities may include swinging in a hammock, balancing on beams, and brushing or stroking and are selected based on each child's sensory needs. Despite considerable acceptance and practice of these therapies by professionals in some countries, there is little evidence to suggest that sensory integration therapies are effective for children with autism (see 'Looking at evidence' in Chapter 10).

ANXIETY

We are all programmed to feel anxious when we are under threat or in danger. Physiological changes such as an increased heart rate, tremors and sweating are part of the so-called 'fight or flight' response when our lives are threatened. Even though we no longer have to respond to life-threatening situations on a day-to-day basis, there are still activities in everyday life that can induce anxiety, such as speaking in public, heights, or certain animals and insects.

Developmentally, there are normal stages that include a component of anxiety, including stranger wariness, during the first year of life. During the toddler and preschool years there are some well-known situations that cause anxiety but these fears usually fade as the child gets older. Two of these are 'fear of the dark' and separation anxiety. Many children also experience a phase of being scared of dressed-up characters. During the toddler and preschool years anxiety is common in children with autism.

Jane and Todd both experienced anxiety during their toddler/preschool years. Todd became very quiet and avoided interacting with people other than his mother and father. This made it difficult for Jessica to leave him with anyone aside from his dad, who worked long hours. Jane showed her anxiety by struggling and needing to be forcibly removed from the car and dragged into the preschool on arrival at the child care centre. Whether this was due to separation anxiety or anxiety about other aspects of the child care was not clear.

IDENTIFYING ANXIETY

It is hard to be sure in young children (and in older children who do not communicate) whether their behaviour is underpinned by anxiety. Sometimes anxiety will seem likely once you have identified the trigger but, if not, it is still good to ask yourself whether your child could be anxious about something.

Some things that create anxiety are more recognisable and acceptable than others. Most people understand a fear of spiders, for example, even at an extreme level. Children with autism can have longer and stronger anxiety responses to well-recognised triggers and can also have anxious responses to unusual triggers.

Our anxiety profile also changes over time. This could be due to sensory perception changes, which might affect how we react over time to different foods or sounds (see also the sections on fussy eating in regard to taste and sensory problems) or because we have learnt that things we were afraid of won't really hurt us.

MANAGING ANXIETY

The first step to managing anxiety is to work out what is actually causing it. If the trigger is an essential part of everyday life, like learning to separate from a parent upon arriving at child care, then trying to avoid the situation won't be possible. If the trigger is avoidable, like going to the supermarket, then avoidance can be a reasonable option, at least in the short term.

In toddlers and preschool children, the best way to manage anxiety is mainly by soothing them and providing reassurance. These actions can be gradually withdrawn while offering positive feedback and rewards for coping. For separation anxiety, if your child is upset because you are leaving, then you should stay and reassure them that everything will be all right. After a while you should leave as planned. The people who remain with your child should continue to soothe and reassure them. As your child is settling they should be offered something interesting and engaging to do.

Giving your child information about likely events in a way they can understand can also be helpful, especially if they like structure and are less anxious when things are more predictable. You could let your child know, using words or pictures, the steps that will unfold when they arrive at their child care and what you will stay for. For example, you might tell them or show them that you will stay while they put their bag in the rack and wash their hands and then you will say goodbye. You can also let them know what will happen during the day and that you will be back to pick them up after their last activity. You may want to leave them for shorter periods initially and pick them up after lunch, for example, gradually increasing the time they spend at child care.

Introducing change at a slow enough rate to manage your child's anxiety may take some time and patience, but the ultimate goal is important and worthwhile. Sticking with a plan is important; you may be able to move through stages quickly or you may have to break activities down into even smaller steps. It is also important to remember that there will be some day-to-day variation, with your child being more anxious on some days than on others. Children with autism also sometimes suddenly stop responding to something with anxiety or start being anxious about something entirely different, which means you need to be flexible. For some children, anxious behaviour will slowly decrease indicating they are less anxious and more able to cope. For others, the behaviour will continue at a high intensity and then suddenly stop. As described in Table 2, it is important that all parents and carers agree on the approach you plan to instigate, and that everyone acts consistently. Professional support from child care staff or from other professionals can be very helpful to support you through this process, monitor your child's progress, and assist with decisions about any changes to the plan that may be needed. Additional interventions are available for older children (see Chapter 9).

BITING, HITTING AND KICKING

Biting, hitting and kicking are common behaviours in toddlers and preschool children. They are said to be 'externalising' because the child has turned an emotion or thought into a physical action that affects others. Such behaviours are more common in younger children because other coping strategies involve more sophisticated abilities, like being able to describe how you feel and think about solutions. For children with autism, understanding and communicating about their thoughts and feelings is particularly difficult.

Although these behaviours are common in toddlers and preschool children, they are socially unacceptable and they can create problems at many levels. If your child bites, hits or kicks other children or adults you are likely to hear about it from the child care or educational facility that your child attends, as well as from other parents. Your child may be avoided by other children, reducing their opportunity for social contact. You may even find that other parents are avoiding you. This, therefore, is an issue that needs to be prioritised. Again, it will need agreed management by all the adults who are involved in your child's care.

The same principles apply in managing this behaviour as to other unwanted behaviours (see Table 2 in Chapter 5). A common trigger is a situation in which your child did not understand what was happening and reacted out of frustration. It could be that your child missed an opportunity to join in or that another child acted in a way that upset them. Improving communication will be a major part of the management approach. An adult may need to be there when these problems arise and advice from a speech therapist may be needed to help with communication strategies.

Your child could be hitting out because another child is interfering with an autism-specific behaviour, like taking something that is an important part of one of their special interests. Here it is important to work with staff at the child care setting so that they understand the trigger in the context of your child and can work with the other children to minimise disruptions that cause your child distress. At the same time the staff will work with your child to model alternative responses and to develop a plan with their early intervention worker about the autism-specific behaviour.

Your child may be responding to being bullied. If you suspect bullying you need to discuss this with the adult carers present and seek their help to assess whether bullying is taking place and how to manage it. Most child care settings and preschools will have procedures in place to promote positive social interaction among children and deal with negative social behaviour like bullying. It is also important to think about ways to help your child minimise opportunities for bullying and to teach them non-aggressive responses like walking away when someone annoys them (see also chapters 7 and 9 for a discussion of bullying when children are older). Children at this age are unlikely to have much understanding of the effect of their behaviour on other people, including other children. Learning this is an important part of the socialisation of children and may be particularly difficult for children with autism. In the toddler and preschool-age group, encouraging pro-social behaviour for all children and rules about anti-social behaviour are likely to be the most effective strategies.

It is also important to directly address biting, hitting or kicking as a response to anger. If it is not possible to decrease the anger in a timely way, then your child needs to be encouraged to adopt a more socially acceptable response, like yelling or stomping their feet. The support of a professional with experience in behaviour management will be needed.

> Todd had an episode of kicking when he first attended child care. This was noted to happen in the afternoon when his learning support aide was not available. The child care staff watched Todd more closely after this happened and noticed that he kicked a child when the child tried to take away one of his vintage cars, which his mum had

told them was his special interest. The child care worker spoke with Todd's early intervention professionals and his mum and it was decided that Todd's special interest would be explained to all the children, that they would be encouraged to talk to him about it but also told not to take his cars away. Todd, with the assistance of his aide, was encouraged to allow other children to sit with him while he played with his vintage cars.

IRRITABILITY

Irritability is a very non-specific behaviour, which can be worrying for you as a parent. When a newborn is irritable, parents get used to working with limited information. They learn to identify the type of irritability their child is exhibiting and link it to a particular need, or work through the three or four things they can change that might be the cause, like hunger, a dirty nappy, tiredness or discomfort. As your child gets older, they may be irritable due to more complicated feelings, like boredom, loneliness or lack of attention.

In autism, irritability of unidentifiable cause can be a more persistent problem. The reason for irritability can be harder to identify because of the difficulties communicating, or because your child has more difficulty understanding or describing how they are feeling.

Irritability may also be linked to physical states that can be more common in autism. One is hunger or iron deficiency that can result from fussy eating or a chosen dietary modification. Others include a lack of sleep or constipation. It could also be that because of a specific routine or fixed behaviour, like wearing a winter jacket even when it is hot or playing with water until extremely wet, your child could be exposed to a range of physical discomforts which, in turn, may cause them to respond with non-specific behaviour. It could also be because of an unusual sensory sensitivity, such as the feeling of certain clothing or clothing labels on the skin.

In toddlers and preschool children, the approach to irritability is to assess the cause by running through possible physical and sensory triggers. If possible physical causes like sleep, diet, constipation and sensory issues have been excluded or remedied, then communication strategies are key so that your child can share their needs with you. Professional help will be required.

TOILET-RELATED BEHAVIOURS

During the toddler and preschool years, children in many societies are trained to control their bladder and bowel so they can use toilet facilities. The age of achieving this behaviour varies widely. As a general rule, daytime training comes before night-time dryness.

For children with autism, any of the behaviours required for successful toilet-training can be delayed or more difficult. The strategies normally used to encourage toilet-training may also take longer to work or may be unsuitable for your child (see Resources at the end of the chapter). Most importantly, the readiness to begin toilet-training may not appear at the usual time. This can be frustrating because toilet-training may be a prerequisite of some child care and educational settings.

Two main patterns emerge when toilet-training a child with autism. It can all go to plan, but later than usual, with the use of special strategies for communication. You may need to use some of the devices that are available to assist with toilet-training. The classic version is the bell and pad alarm system for night-time wetting, with the unpleasant (often for the whole family) experience of being wakened to trigger your child to stop weeing and go to the toilet. These approaches have about an 80 per cent success rate. More modern versions are now available and some can be adapted for daytime use. These devices are available from your pharmacy, but it is best to talk with your doctor and early intervention professionals first, if possible. These sorts of approaches are also ideally reinforced with a positive reward cycle, such as a chart to show successful nights or days and a small reward for achieving goals. You may also have access to services for children with a developmental disability who have problems with continence.

Alternatively, your child may have autism-specific behaviours that are slowing down the toilet-training process. This can include a specific resistance to using the toilet, heightened sensory issues during weeing and pooing that make the experience more unpleasant for your child, and concern about using different toilets.

John's parents noticed he went to the same place at home behind the sofa when he did a poo. They worked with their therapist and started a program which involved showing him his toilet card and prompting him to tap it while moving quickly to the toilet as soon as he started going behind the sofa. If he used the toilet they made a big fuss and gave him his favourite action–response toy as a reward. In addition, Sue and Mike continued to take John to the toilet regularly, always using the toilet card and rewarding John for using the toilet. Eventually John started to bring them the card when he wanted to go to the toilet and tapped it to indicate what he wanted. At home he also just took himself off to the bathroom sometimes and could use the toilet fairly reliably, although he needed help to wipe his bottom after a poo and needed prompting to wash his hands. At preschool John also learnt to go to the toilet when all the children went. His early intervention teacher set up a series of photos showing each stage of the process for John to follow and showed the preschool staff how to use the pictures to help John learn to do it by himself. Over several months he learnt to urinate, do a poo and wash his hands with fewer and fewer prompts until he was able to do everything independently except for wiping his bottom after a poo. After six months at preschool John no longer needed to wear pull-ups (nappies).

CONSTIPATION

There are very rarely medical reasons for problems with toilet-training. The most common problem is constipation (hard to pass or infrequent poos or both) which should be managed in discussion with your doctor. As a rule, you should increase water intake, increase high fibre foods including fruit and vegetables (which is not always easy at this age), and increase daily exercise. If these steps fail then it is best to use an osmotic laxative, one that draws fluid into the bowel to soften the poo, to re-establish a pooing routine. In some situations constipation can become more severe and can appear as liquid stools if the rectum, the lowest part of the bowel, is so clogged that only 'overflow' poo is able to come out. This most commonly occurs following a viral illness, during which your child can become dehydrated and prone to constipation. If your child has tried to poo and this has caused pain and sometimes bleeding, your child may then decide that it is best not to poo, which can create a cycle of 'holding on'. This needs to be broken. Seek help from your doctor if you suspect this could be a problem. Early intervention professionals with experience in working with children with autism will also be able to support you and your child.

OTHER POO- AND WEE-RELATED BEHAVIOURS

Some children with autism also develop unwanted behaviours related to pooing and weeing, including smearing and throwing poo. These behaviours need to be managed as a matter of priority as they are socially unacceptable and create health hazards. As with other behaviours, it is good to think through the factors that come before the behaviour and to try to identify any possible triggers. These might include attention seeking, sensory stimulation or boredom. Once possible triggers are identified, address these to reduce the incidence of the behaviour. The fact that people tend to react very strongly to this sort of behaviour may be making it really interesting for your child and more likely that they will do it again. You may also want to consider strategies to prevent the behaviour in the short term, such as barrier methods (e.g. your child wearing bib and brace overalls) while other approaches to coping in more socially acceptable ways are developed. Helpful strategies also include the prevention of constipation to decrease the focus on pooing, and rewards for putting poo in the right place, that is, in the toilet.

MASTURBATION

Masturbation is not uncommon and is a normal part of development in the preschool years. There is no need to intervene, unless masturbation is causing a physical problem, or occurring in public, in which case you need to teach your child that it is a behaviour for a private place. If masturbation continues to occur frequently in public settings, it should be addressed in the same way as other unwanted behaviours (see Chapter 5). For further information about masturbation see 'Sexuality and relationships' in Chapter 9.

DIET AND NUTRITION

FUSSY OR PICKY EATING

Lots of children are fussy eaters. This behaviour is most common in the toddler and preschool years. Fussiness can be about texture (children eating only crunchy foods or only soft, smooth food), taste or colour (children only eating white or specific coloured foods). Some children can be concerned about how the food is served, wanting all the different foods on the plate to be separate and some even want different foods to be served on different plates. Theories about food fussiness include biological reasons, like heightened taste awareness at a younger age, especially for bitter flavours. Others relate to autonomy and control as part of psychological development, and note that oral intake is one of the few things that a child can control in the early years (see Resources at the end of the chapter). Children with autism have fussy or picky eating habits more often than other children.

Parents may worry that their child is not getting adequate nutrition, and can also be concerned that having very specific likes and dislikes about food may add to problems with social engagement, as people often come together around food. Feeding your child is also a primary driver for any parent or carer, so it can be emotionally challenging if a child isn't seen to be eating well. Any concern you have is likely to be compounded by comments made by others, such as family and friends. Unfortunately, your child's eating is one of those topics that people feel they can comment on, as well as offer well-meaning advice.

If you live in a high-income country it is unlikely that your child will become undernourished because of food fussiness to a level that could impair their growth and development. Generally, we eat more than is needed to maintain growth and development. Many foods are also fortified with essential vitamins and other nutrients to a level that makes it easier to ensure children reach their daily requirements.

Iron is one dietary requirement that can be hard to get enough of for non-red meat eaters. An inadequate intake of iron can lead to anaemia, which in turn can change behaviour by making your child more tired and irritable, and also less interested in eating. Iron is most easily obtained from breast milk for the very young and then from meat, because iron delivered by these sources is more easily absorbed. This means even a small amount of red meat is sufficient. There are also other foods rich in iron, and tablet and syrup preparations of iron are available if needed. If your child has no meat intake, either because of your choice or their food fussiness, then it is advisable to speak with your doctor. A blood test may be needed to see if they would benefit from an iron supplement (see Resources at the end of the chapter).

> Jane was a fussy eater when she was a toddler, preferring pale foods such as white bread, chicken breast, mashed potato and rice. She was reluctant to try new things and would not eat any green or yellow food and only ate puréed pale fruit. She also would not tolerate her food

mixed up and would not eat it if it was touching other food on her plate.

You may also have read that gluten, a protein found in wheat, and casein, a protein found in milk, can cause autism or make behaviours worse (more on this on the next page). This could be adding to your concerns, especially if your child is particularly fond of white foods, including bread and milk, or soft textures, such as yoghurt and custard. You may wonder if a certain food is causing your child problems and that is why they are refusing it.

Food allergy and food intolerance are increasingly reported problems. There is a chance your child will have one of these, however they don't usually show up as food refusal. If you have noticed a pattern that links certain types of food ingestion to vomiting or diarrhoea or behaviours that suggest your child is in pain, or your child has had skin reactions or breathing problems after eating a food, then you should discuss this with your doctor. Most children grow out of food allergies during the preschool years (see Resources at the end of the chapter).

Your child may also be gagging during meals, which is very distressing to watch. Gagging is a normal reflex that is triggered when objects touch the back of your mouth or tongue. We gag to prevent dangerous objects entering our airway. Gagging can lead to vomiting. Some children (and adults) gag more readily than others and this is sometimes called a hypersensitive gag reflex. Being worried about something or being agitated can heighten your gag reflex or trigger it. If gagging is only occurring in association with food fussiness behaviours then it is best to think of it as a symptom of that behaviour and to address the food fussiness not the gagging behaviour directly. If gagging is occurring when your child is eating calmly or if it is associated with coughing and choking then you should discuss this with your doctor.

As a parent, it is best not to feel guilty about the way your child eats. It might be necessary to consciously minimise your own anxiety about your child's eating to be sure you are not acting in a way that could lead to more, rather than less, fussiness. Like other behaviours, it is good to seek professional advice about this to both guide your attempts at behaviour management but also to provide support, as it will be challenging for you and your child's other carers.

CHANGING FUSSY EATING BEHAVIOURS

It is important to 'pick your battles' and only address one unwanted behaviour at a time. So if you are reassured that your child is getting adequate nutrition for growth and development you can leave their eating habits until later if other things are a priority. If you feel that your child's eating is your main concern at present, then we know that children need multiple trials of a new taste before they will accept it. The approaches used to improve eating behaviours include praising or rewarding success, ignoring failure, and building on success (see Table 2 in Chapter 5), and only change one thing at a time when trying to modify a specific eating behaviour. For example, introduce new foods one at a time and in very small amounts.

To introduce different tastes and textures, offer foods with a similar taste or texture to the foods your child already likes. For example, if they like crunchy food such as potato chips and you would like to broaden their repertoire, then pick something that is the next step along that they are not eating, such as potatoes cut smaller than usual and baked until crisp. If there are some food groups that you would like your child to eat that are currently not eaten at all, such as fruit, then select a fruit that has the most similar consistency or colour to the foods they already like. If your child only eats white food, peel an apple and offer that raw if they like crunchy food, or cooked if they like soft food. When introducing new foods only offer very small amounts, with a reward or praise for eating the amount that is offered. If the new food was eaten then you can serve slightly more of that food the second time, and so on. If the food was not eaten, continue offering the same very small amount until it is.

Probably the least concerning, but perhaps the most irritating, are food behaviours about wanting food to be separated. This becomes a problem when eating outside the home when food separation is not possible. While working toward minimising this unwanted behaviour at home, it is reasonable to take food when eating out to avoid all the other problems that are likely to follow from food being served in a different way. If this is your child's only fussy eating behaviour then it is fine to try to modify it. If it is one of many, then leave this one until last. The priority has to be nutrition and ensuring your child is getting enough of a range of foods for growth and development. This might be quite a small selection of food. Many people are fussy eaters and have a limited range of foods they like.

> Jane's parents followed the suggestions their early intervention professional gave them (similar advice is now available on websites like the ones listed in the Resources at the end of this chapter) and over one year Jane increased the range of foods she was eating so that they were no longer worried. Using the same sort of approaches, they gradually increased the foods she ate during her primary school years. Given all the other things that were happening in their lives they never focused on her preference not to mix different foods. At the end of secondary school she still preferred to keep her foods separated but could tolerate some meals that combined foods when eating out, especially at her favourite fast food restaurant.

GLUTEN AND CASEIN FREE DIET

If you have heard that gluten, which is found in wheat, and casein, which is found in milk, can cause or worsen autism you may think about trying a gluten and casein free diet. Todd's parents did. It is important to know that this theory about gluten and casein causing or exacerbating autism has existed since the 1990s but a causal link has never been proven. A gluten and casein free diet has also never been shown to improve autism or its commonly associated problems (see Resources at the end of the chapter). There are possible harms of a gluten and casein free diet, including bone health because dairy products, which are eliminated in the diet, are a good source of calcium. Gluten and casein free products often cost more and being on a special diet will mean that at social gatherings, like birthday parties, your child won't be able to join in social activities around food as easily. The diet will also add complexity if your child is already fussy about food. This is a particular concern if your child already has a very limited diet and you are considering further restricting the range of foods they eat.

> Todd's parents tried a gluten and casein free diet during the preschool years. They let their doctor know they were doing this and she referred them to a dietician so they could get good advice and support while Todd was on the diet, as well as monitor Todd's growth and nutrition. Todd remained well but his parents weren't sure if the diet had made a difference to the behaviours they had heard it would change, like his interest in other children. Jessica thought it had reduced his irritability and anxiety but his dad Joseph didn't agree. They decided to stop the diet when he went to school to make going to parties and lunch box packing easier. Jessica noticed that reintroducing gluten and casein in Todd's diet wasn't associated with a significant change in his behaviour, even though he was starting school, which was new and different.

VITAMIN AND NUTRITIONAL SUPPLEMENTS

There has been interest in dietary supplementation with vitamins and omega-3 fatty acids as possible ways to improve the core features of autism. Unless your child has a vitamin deficiency then there is no need to give vitamin and other dietary supplements. In some cases, excess amounts can cause harm. If you are planning to commence a dietary supplement it is worth discussing this with your doctor and ensuring you are monitoring for positive and negative outcomes (see Resources at the end of the chapter).

PICA

Pica is a fancy word used to describe eating non-food substances. It is not uncommon among toddlers in particular, especially eating playdough, as John did. For some children, eating non-food substances is a concern, either because of what they eat potentially posing risks to their health, or because of their focus on this behaviour and the secondary behaviours that occur when their eating is stopped. In toddlers and preschool children it can be hard to assess the motivation for a behaviour, but the eating of non-food substances may be a compulsion, which means that it is an act your child will feel they have to complete. Addressing this is not straightforward. Removing the opportunity is ideal and easier if only certain non-food substances are eaten. Any positive outcomes from the act of eating non-food substances should be minimised. Certainly eating non-food items attracts a lot of attention, and needs to if there is a risk of harm because of the ingestion. If, however, there is no risk of harm then minimising attention may assist. The behaviour should be managed in the same way as other problem behaviours (see Table 2 in Chapter 5). Again, working as a team with other carers and assistance from professionals are both important. Medical help should be sought if there is an acute or longer-term health risk such as ingesting heavy metal from picking and swallowing flakes of lead-based paint.

> Because John was at no risk from eating small amounts of playdough, this behaviour was ignored when he was out and playdough was around. Playdough was not available for him to use at home. Over a year John's playdough eating behaviour stopped.

ABSCONDING

During the toddler and preschool years children with autism may run away. See Chapter 8 for more information about absconding.

IF SKILLS ARE LOST

The toddler years are a time of rapid change. If your child had skills and then lost them, you should seek medical advice as a matter of some urgency. See the section 'If skills are lost' in Chapter 3 for more information about skill loss in autism, including diagnosing it and necessary investigations.

GETTING READY FOR SCHOOL

Your early intervention professionals and the teachers at your child's new school will assist you and your child with the transition to school. The types of things that will help with your child's transition are assisting your child to learn appropriate skills as well as you and your child's current professionals working with the new school so they have a good understanding of your child's skills and needs. It is important that you and your child visit the new school and that your child learns more about the school and what to expect through visual supports, such as stories and pictures. Remember, visual suppports must be at a level your child understands.

TELLING YOUR CHILD ABOUT THEIR DIFFERENCES

As you get ready for school it is worth thinking about how and when you will discuss with your child that they are different to other children. The timing of this will vary depending on your child's level of understanding and communication. We mention this here because a greater awareness of autism within the broader community has been matched in children and young people. It is not uncommon to hear children use old and new diagnostic terms for autism when they are talking about their peers. This means that your child may have their differences pointed out to them in the school grounds and be labelled, correctly or incorrectly, by their classmates.

It is best to think about differences, rather than diagnoses, when talking with your child. We are all different, with myriad abilities, interests, temperaments and personalities. If you begin with the differences that are most evident and discuss how others might see them, then this can also be part of providing suggestions for how your child can cope if they are teased in the playground or having difficulties in the classroom (see Resources below).

RESOURCES

Sleep in toddlers and preschoolers

> http://raisingchildren.net.au/sleep/toddlers_sleep.html

> http://raisingchildren.net.au/articles/preschoolers_sleep_nutshell.html

Sleep in autism

> http://raisingchildren.net.au/articles/autism_spectrum_disorder_sleep_difficulties.html

> www.psychology.org.au/inpsych/2014/april/rinehart/

> http://pediatrics.aappublications.org/content/134/2/298.long

> www.researchautism.net/research-autism-our-research/research-autism-projects-completed/snuggledown-weighted-blankets

www.bmj.com/content/345/bmj.e6664

Auditory integration training (AIT) systematic review

http://onlinelibrary.wiley.com/doi/10.1002/14651858.CD003681.pub3/abstract

Sensory integration therapy evidence summaries

www.crd.york.ac.uk/crdweb/ShowRecord.asp?ID=12012026826

http://effectivehealthcare.ahrq.gov/index.cfm/search-for-guides-reviews-and-reports/?productid=651&pageaction=displayproduct

Toilet-training

http://raisingchildren.net.au/articles/toilet_training.html

Iron deficiency and improving iron intake

www.nhlbi.nih.gov/health/health-topics/topics/ida/

www.schn.health.nsw.gov.au/parents-and-carers/fact-sheets/ways-to-boost-iron-intake

Food allergy and intolerance

http://raisingchildren.net.au/articles/recognising_allergies.html/context/949

Approaches to fussy eating

www.autismspeaks.org/family-services/health-and-wellness/nutrition/seven-ways-help-picky-eater-autism

http://raisingchildren.net.au/articles/fussy_eating.html/context/729

Summary of evidence about gluten and casein free diet as an intervention

www.crd.york.ac.uk/crdweb/ShowRecord.asp?LinkFrom=OAI&ID=12010003744#.VC441CmSzpd

Other nutritional therapies

www.thecochranelibrary.com/details/browseReviews/579405/Autistic-spectrum-disorder.html?page=1 to find systematic reviews about omega-3 fatty acids and combined vitamin B6/magnesium therapy

Telling your child about their differences

www.autism.org.uk/about-autism/all-about-diagnosis/diagnosis-the-process-for-children/recently-diagnosed-children.aspx

www.autism.org.uk/products/leaflets/after-diagnosis.aspx

www.iidc.indiana.edu/?pageId=362 has information and a list of some books you may find useful

CHAPTER 7

THE PRIMARY SCHOOL YEARS

Children attend primary (junior) school from early childhood to the early teenage years. During these years your child will grow, mature and be challenged as the expectations of school increase and the relationships with friends become more complex.

GOING TO SCHOOL

Luke Jackson, a young man with Asperger's syndrome explains in the book *Freaks, Geeks and Asperger Syndrome. A user guide to adolescence*: 'For some people school is like fitting a square peg in a round hole. For me at the moment the hole (school) has changed its shape slightly to accommodate me and the square peg (me) has tried to soften its edges. So a better description would be a rounded square trying to fit itself into a circle with sticky out bits.'[1]

Today there is growing understanding and acceptance of the idea that we need to adapt the school environment to accommodate children with autism and other developmental problems and disabilities, as well as teach children with autism the specific skills they need to be able to participate in school. However, turning this understanding into a reality varies across schools and school systems and each child's experience will be different.

Transition to school is known to be a stressful time and a period when new problems can appear or pre-existing difficulties or unwanted behaviours can become more marked in children with autism.

> During Todd's transition to school his behaviour became very rigid and ritualistic. He insisted on carrying model vintage cars from his collection in each hand and would frequently hold them up to his face and spin the wheels which made it very difficult for him to do anything else. He would only wear one layer of clothing and demanded that in any room he was in at school all the cupboard doors had to be closed and the tissues tucked into their boxes. If there were tissues poking out of the box or if cupboard doors were ajar he could not attend to anything else. The school psychologist wondered if this could be obsessive compulsive disorder (OCD) (see 'Anxiety disorders' in Chapter 9 for more information about OCD) but his paediatrician suggested his behaviours were an increase of some pre-existing autism behaviours and most likely related to anxiety because of transition to school. A period of observation was agreed and during the next six months Todd's unwanted behaviours decreased.

CHOOSING A PRIMARY SCHOOL

In most countries there are government or public schools and non-government or private schools. Schools in these sectors may be primary (junior) only (4 to 12/13 years of age), secondary (high) school only (12/13 to 18 years of age) or both (4 to 18 years). Sometimes there are separate middle or intermediate schools catering for children between primary and secondary school (11 to 14 years of age). In some countries there are also special schools that cater specifically for children with disabilities. These may be general (catering for children with all disabilities), or specialised (catering for children with a specific disability such as deafness or autism). In many countries there is an increasing trend towards educating all children in regular schools and legislation often exists to ensure children with additional educational needs are accommodated. Home-schooling is also an option in many countries.

Choosing a primary school for your child is likely to be confronting and stressful for a variety of reasons. You will be realising that your child will need ongoing additional support to cope in a regular classroom, or may need more support than a mainstream setting can offer. Understanding your child's abilities and support needs is an important part of making this decision. Having information about your child's communication and cognitive abilities is an integral part of this decision-making. It is also essential for teachers and schools to adapt the environment and curriculum to your child to cater for any additional needs. If you have been given several options, then choosing the right school for your child can be very challenging. While choice increases the possibility of getting the right fit for your child, there are likely to be pros and cons associated with each option, which need to be weighed up.

Don't be afraid to ask for help from the professionals you are working with or to let the schools you are talking to know about the processes or choices that you are finding hard. Having said that, although professional guidance should assist with decision-making, you may sometimes get conflicting advice, which creates a problem in itself. In one study, early intervention professionals were more likely to recommend enrolment in a regular classroom, while education professionals recommended special school/class placement for the same child, with conflicting advice particularly common when children were considered 'borderline' in terms of their intellectual ability.[2]

It is probably most important that a school has a positive climate. The school culture is determined in large part by the school principal and their leadership. You will be able to tell before you enrol your child whether the school has a welcoming 'can do' approach. It is best to avoid schools that don't, if at all possible.

Schools should have the capacity to provide an individual program for your child (more on this below). However, you don't want them to only focus on the changes that your child needs to make to fit into the system. The school should be flexible and have the ability to make changes to its environment too, like the provision of sanctuary spaces or lunchtime clubs. They should have a program in place so all students in the school know about autism. A good school will also work proactively with you. Making a school 'autism friendly' will not only ensure improved educational and social outcomes for your child, it will benefit the whole school.

> Jane was lucky to have a local primary school with some experience with children with autism and because the school was in a rural area the classes were small. The principal and her teachers knew she needed visual supports to help her make sense of the world even though she talked quite well. For example, they provided easy-to-understand structures and routines by setting up daily picture schedules showing the timetable.

In reality, the sort of school your child is enrolled in will vary depending on your geography, government policy and the school system of the day, as well as your child's characteristics and your financial circumstances.

> Jane had no choice because of where she lived whereas Todd's parents could choose between the public and

private system. For both Jane and Todd there was agreement from all professionals about attending a regular school.

When deciding on a school for John, his parents weighed up the advantages of inclusion in a regular classroom, particularly the opportunity to learn social skills from peers, against the academic and social expectations and sensory demands of regular classrooms. John attended a special school. His class included five other children ranging in age from five to eight with moderate to severe intellectual disability. Two of the other children in John's class also had autism. Classes in the school were staffed with a teacher and a teacher's aide (assistant). Some of the children in the school had physical disabilities too. Each child in John's class had an individual learning program.

TEACHERS

Teachers are a vital part of any school. In most countries, primary schools teach a national curriculum with universal assessment of children. Teachers in primary schools must have an in-depth understanding of their national curriculum, and are increasingly expected to be able to assess the academic capacity and needs of the range of diverse learners in their classroom and develop ways to adjust the regular curriculum to enable all the students in their class to participate.

Your child's teacher should have a thorough knowledge of the characteristics of autism and of your child. In-depth knowledge about autism-specific programs and interventions may not be a realistic expectation to have for every teacher, however specialist staff, who can offer support to develop, implement and evaluate individual programs for your child, should be accessible. With this knowledge and assistance they will be able to cater for your child's needs, regardless of the type of educational placement. You can ask whether school staff have access to ongoing professional development about the inclusion of diverse learners and children with autism in particular. One parent reported '... it has been my experience that unless the classroom teacher has some experience and/or training, the child begins the year with a series of crises and the teacher gains experience by managing these problems'.[3] Fortunately knowledge about best teaching practices and classroom approaches for children with additional needs is constantly growing, but this also poses a challenge for teachers who need ongoing training and support to keep up with developments.

If your child is in a regular classroom, like Jane, Todd and Siew, their teacher will be facing a number of challenges in order to ensure that the inclusive arrangements bring maximum benefits to your child, to you and to the school community as a whole.

In the same way typical children progress at school, children with autism progress through the curricula at a rate right for their level of ability and the skill of their teachers. Children with autism are more likely to have a scatter of skills, for example be good at word recognition but have difficulty understanding the meaning of the words. There is also the possibility that children with autism develop at uneven rates, so academic progress may appear to plateau or even regress at times.

INDIVIDUAL PLANNING

Prior to commencing school, whether specialist or regular, an individualised plan that takes account of your child's current needs and strengths, and sets out realistic, functional, prioritised, measurable long- and short-term goals and details strategies to be implemented to meet those goals will be developed. The plan will include the timeframe for implementation, review and revision of the goals, and describe both *what* your child will be taught (content) and *how* your child will be taught (process).

Transition to school will be the focus of your child's plan in the year before they start and will include consideration of the environmental changes and adaptations needed to make the move from preschool or early intervention seamless and positive. In some, but not all, countries, provision of an individual plan is mandated in law, although there is variability and you may find that the focus of individual planning is on the curriculum, rather than the strengths and needs of your child. In other words, the plan for your child documents the adjustments required in the national curriculum to accommodate your child, rather than addresses your child's characteristics, strengths and needs (see Resources at the end of the chapter). The most effective individual program for your child will include both.

> At school John was assessed with regard to his current skills and what skills he needed to develop. Sue and Mike were told that they would be given an appointment before the end of the first term to come into the school and meet with John's teacher, Janet, to discuss his assessment and the goals the school planned to work on with John. Janet noted John's very limited receptive and expressive communication. He understood some simple verbal phrases such as 'toilet', 'let's go', 'eating' and 'playground'. He was usually able to follow some simple one-step instructions that he was familiar with as long as he was calm. These instructions usually consisted of one or two words accompanied by showing John what the teacher wanted him to understand. He experienced great difficulties with transitions between activities and became anxious and sometimes quite distressed during these times. He continued to be non-verbal and took Janet or his learning support aide by the hand without eye contact and tugged them in the direction of what he was unable to reach for himself. He made a particular sound as a form of protest. Janet incorporated his visual communication system into the system used in the classroom. She had already set up a visually based communication system in the classroom for the other students so this was not difficult.

School staff and some of the other students used pictures to communicate with John, although the other students tended to stop trying when John didn't respond. Janet planned to focus on teaching him to use his pictures to initiate communication at school, rather than leading adults by the hand when he wanted something. She decided many of John's unwanted behaviours were due to his frustration at not being able to communicate.

Janet also noted that John had restricted interests and that one of these was playdough which he would play with repetitively and eat. He also showed an interest in the telephone directory and would flip through it. He had a set of about twenty brightly coloured small books in the classroom. Janet gave him a few of these at a time, which he flipped through in a particular order. She noted that when he was engaged with his special interests he became intensely preoccupied with them, followed his strict routines and often had difficulty moving on to the next activity. Janet used John's special interests to teach him new skills. For example she put the playdough in clear containers with tight lids in a special box on a high shelf and showed John how to ask for what he wanted by showing her a picture of the playdough and signing 'help'. Similarly, she prompted him to sign 'help' to get the lid off the playdough containers. She had different coloured playdough and taught him to match the colours. She gave him something else to chew on while he was playing with the playdough which reduced the number of times he put it into his mouth.

Collaborative proactive planning and preparation by a team ensures that strategies are in place to help your child cope with this major change, to participate in school and to learn. The development, implementation and review of the plan should involve you, all relevant professionals working with your child/family, teachers from your child's school and, where possible, your child.

There is no one intervention plan or defined support pathway that will meet the needs of all children with autism, primarily because of the wide individual variability among students with autism. For example, John's needs would be different to Todd's.

If your child has any health issues, like epilepsy, you will want to know that school staff can manage this problem as well as you can, just as John's parents did. Your child will need a plan for usual care and also for care in the event of an acute problem, like a seizure, that the school staff can follow. This plan will need to be developed by your doctor and shared with the school. The school will need to arrange any special training that is needed for staff because of your child's health issue. The plan of action followed by staff at the school will be the same as the plan you would follow at home.

WHAT INTERVENTIONS TO EXPECT AT SCHOOL

It is unlikely that a comprehensive autism-specific learning-based program will be implemented in your child's school in its exact form. What is more likely is that the school will incorporate some elements of some programs into their process and practice for your child. Implementation of autism-specific learning-based programs is more likely in special schools and support classes than in mainstream classrooms, but all aspects of implemented programs will depend on the expertise and experience of the staff in the school. In mainstream educational settings, it is reasonable to expect a range of relevant autism-specific strategies to be implemented to match the strengths and needs of your child.

COMMUNICATION

Increasing the ability to communicate in the school setting is usually the core need for a child with autism. If your child is in a regular school they could be offered one or more of a range of recommended strategies to improve their communication. The type of intervention used should take into account what is best suited to your child's needs, as well as your preferences and staff expertise. It should also have specific goals in mind.

The question you will want to ask is: 'What strategies are likely to be the most effective given the available resources, and my child's age and stage of development?'

Remember, a communication strategy must be tailored to the level of symbolism your child understands and will work best if your child is communicating about something they are interested in.

> Jessica explained that she had given up asking children around to play with Todd. Together the teacher and Todd's parents decided that a social communication program would be great for Todd at home and at school. His teacher said she would make sure consistent approaches were used in the classroom for all the students, some others of whom she believed would also benefit from social communication skills development. The program incorporated vintage cars and a turn-taking game.

Strategies that capitalise on your child's visual skills can be very helpful. These approaches will show your child, as well as telling them, what is happening or expected and will also give them a way to show you what they may be unable to explain verbally. Visual supports may be used for communication (see also Chapter 5) or to provide order, structure and meaning in the environment (for example, visual schedules which are pictures showing the steps in a task). Technology advances like digital cameras are a great way to create relevant visual supports both easily and relatively cheaply. Social stories, social scripts and comic strip conversations are resources which may be useful in helping children with autism understand social situations. Social stories present visual information (ensure it is at a level your child understands) about situations that your child finds challenging and tell them the way to behave in those situations.

There are also an increasing number of computer and smartphone or tablet programs (apps) available for autism. Some of these are more useful than others so it is important to think critically about what might work best for your child before investing time and money. Using an iPad or tablet can be highly motivating for children and is also socially acceptable (see Resources at the end of the chapter).

CAPITALISING ON SPECIAL INTERESTS

Your child may have special interests in specific things or topics. In the past sometimes this behaviour was discouraged in the belief that special interests interfered with learning. Trying to eliminate special interests takes a lot of time and energy and is usually unsuccessful. Now we believe that these special interests should be harnessed to promote learning by using them as a reward for completing other less preferred activities or by including them in activities.

> John has a chart at school showing him that if he sits on the floor with the other kids for story time he can have his flip books during free time.

> Todd's teacher encouraged him to present to the class at news time about the vintage cars he saw at the weekend. She ensured that all the children, including Todd, knew they had a maximum of five minutes to give their news to the class. She used a timer so they could see how much time they had.

EMOTION RECOGNITION AND REGULATION

Your child may have difficulty recognising and managing emotions in themselves and in other people. Lack of ability to tune in to, or an oversensitivity to the expression of emotions of others, may be an underpinning problem in autism. People vary widely in their ability to read body language and empathise and your child is likely to be less able to do this than most. This, along with an inability to understand that other people have thoughts and feelings that are different to their own (see Chapter 3 for information about theory of mind), is likely to be a major contributing factor to their social difficulties, so it is an important issue to address. Your child may be able to learn to recognise emotional cues in others, but they may need to come to understand this in an intellectual way, rather than the intuitive way that most people use. There are resources available to support emotion recognition that can be incorporated into a program tailored to your child's abilities and needs (see Resources at the end of this chapter).

Your child may also have difficulty understanding and regulating their own feelings of anxiety, anger, sadness and joy. This problem is not limited to children with autism and there are strategies to assist in the recognition of emotions in themselves that are included in interventions for recogising emotion in others. These can then be linked to the types of interventions for behaviour change discussed in Chapter 5 and more specific therapies, for example for anxiety and aggressive behaviour, described in chapters 8 and 10. In this approach the antecedent (or trigger) has two parts: the event and the emotion that was created but was not able to be understood or processed.

SPLINTER AND SAVANT SKILLS

All children with autism have an uneven profile of skill development and some children with autism, about 10 to 25 per cent, have skills that are developed beyond the level expected for their age. These are called splinter or savant skills. The development of these strengths should be incorporated into your child's educational plan, with the goal of developing useful vocational skills in the long term and capitalising on their powerful interests (see Resources at the end of the chapter).

> Todd had prodigious mathematical abilities but difficulties conforming to the usual patterns of mathematical teaching and learning. Before he started preschool, Todd could add and subtract, divide and multiply numbers rapidly in his head. Todd was not taught calculation but worked it out for himself. He sat and manipulated numbers for hours as soon as he learnt to use a pencil. When he walked with Jessica to his grandparents' house, on arrival he would sit and draw all the letterboxes they had passed on the way in their exact order with the numbers on each. In fact, he refused to greet or acknowledge his grandparents until he had drawn all the letterboxes he and his mother had passed. If the number was on the house rather than on the letterbox, he drew the section of the house with the number. At school Todd astonished his teachers with his ability to do mental arithmetic, however he had difficulty in class because number work was based on problem-solving and was also language-based. As he progressed through school, Todd continued to be able to do increasingly complex calculations mentally but he was unable to understand the methods the teacher was teaching to the other children in the class and could not show any 'working'. He just seemed to know the answer and was not able to demonstrate how he had arrived at it.

LEARNING STYLE

Like Todd with his mathematical ability, your child may learn differently to other children. This can occur whether or not your child has a savant skill.

There are many different ways to learn and we all differ in how we learn best. Some people are visual learners while others learn best by listening. We've mentioned this already in regard to the importance of visual opportunities for children with autism who often struggle to understand spoken information. Another difference is whether we learn things in small incremental steps or in chunks or large leaps. Learning or understanding things in chunks can make it difficult for your child to explain how they came to a conclusion, even if the conclusion is right. This can create problems complying with expectations for exams, where the process to the answer is rewarded more than the answer itself. It can also mean that if there is a need for adaptation, because of an error or to move to the next level, it is harder. This type of thinking and learning is demonstrated in the speech of children with autism, who may learn language as chunks rather than by applying linguistic rules to generate novel strings of words.

> Siew learnt to say 'I'm fine, thank you' if people asked him 'How are you?' but he also said 'I'm fine, thank you' when he was asked 'How old are you?'.

Much is known about different learning styles but there are still gaps in how this knowledge is applied to understanding autism and assisting children in school. If you think that your child's learning style is underpinning a difficulty they are having, then discussing it with their teacher is the best first step.

MANAGING SENSORY ISSUES AT SCHOOL

For many children with autism school is a noisy, chaotic environment and on some days they find it hard to cope. By this stage, you will have a good understanding of the sensory issues which are a problem for your child. These could include high-pitched sounds, close contact with other people, or the sensation of wearing shoes. The playground can be particularly difficult. Your child may not recognise the source of their growing anxiety, or may have difficulty communicating what it is. These issues should be discussed with your child's teacher to ensure that strategies are in place to help them cope. Strategies may involve managing the environment, for example ensuring your child has a calm, safe place they can go to if they are feeling overwhelmed and also that they know how to ask for a break.

> Todd found the sound of the buzzer that rang to signal the end of recess or lunchtime distressing until his teacher developed a visual schedule for him showing the times and gave Todd a five-minute warning that the buzzer was about to ring. This enabled Todd to cope with the sound. He also learnt to take deep breaths when he started to feel anxious. When he was having a really bad day, he was allowed to wear headphones which cancelled out environmental sounds.

Involve your child as much as possible to find out what they are experiencing.

> When asked, Todd said, 'The buzzer makes a really bad noise like a dagger going through my head, which hurts a lot. Some days it's worse than others. On bad days I wear my headphones, which makes the buzzer not so bad.'

BULLYING

More than half of all children report being bullied in the school years and bullying is known to be more common amongst children with autism. In this section we focus on bullying in the primary school years as it is important to start as early as possible to prevent bullying and the damaging effects it can have on everyone concerned, but especially for your child. Much of this section will also be relevant to the secondary school years, however bullying issues which are most likely to be prevalent in secondary school are dealt with in Chapter 9. There is growing awareness of the importance of identifying and managing bullying in schools and every school should have a policy and plan for bullying. In addition, there are many excellent web-based resources, some of which are listed at the end of this chapter.

Bullying involves an imbalance of power and can be physical or psychological. Bullying may take the form of verbal aggression (derogatory comments, name-calling and taunting) or physical aggression (hitting, kicking, shoving and spitting). Children may also be socially excluded, however being excluded from a social group might not be very distressing for your child, who may prefer to be on their own anyway. A lack of social skills and not being able to understand someone else's perspective could make your child a target for bullies, especially in the later primary school years. The impact of verbal or physical bullying can be profound and debilitating, however the signs of bullying may not be obvious and even verbally able children may have difficulty communicating with you about it. You may instead notice features that indicate bullying, like changes in your child's behaviour (such as a reluctance to attend school), changes in daily routines (their eating or sleeping habits are suddenly different), a decline in academic performance, increase in emotionally sensitive behaviour and anxiety, or obvious indicators such as torn clothing, damaged books or other items, as well as cuts or bruises. If you notice any of these things do consider if bullying could be taking place.

STRATEGIES TO PREVENT AND MANAGE BULLYING

Schools have a responsibility to keep children safe. The best way to do this is to ensure there is a culture of respect throughout the school. Students and staff should understand what bullying is, that it is not acceptable and that there are consequences. A good school will also celebrate behaviours when children support each other. School staff should be aware of group dynamics and separate known 'trouble-makers'. School policies and processes should include adequate supervision of students at all times and safe ways to report bullying, for example a 'bullying box' where students can report bullying if they fear retaliation. Your child may need to be taught about bullying behaviours, both physical and verbal, and exactly what to do if they are being bullied. A proactive approach to minimise bullying might include developing a 'circle of friends', a group of six to eight children who volunteer to support and include your child. Bullying is more likely to take place in unstructured times such as break time, transition between classes, and before or after school. The school could assist by creating structure at break times, perhaps designating certain areas of the playground for specific activities, such as ball play. Your child may find it easier to take part in these structured activities and avoid areas they find overwhelming, as will other children. An area of the playground could be designated for 'quiet play' or access could be allowed to rooms in the school building, such as the library, during breaks. Staff supervision is still needed to make sure these spaces are safe but should not be done in a way that draws attention to your child. If your child uses public transport to and from school, finding 'travel buddies' may help.

> Once Todd had been at school for two terms his teacher spoke to his parents about her concern that he was having problems interacting with his peers. Todd has a soft monotonous voice and tended to lecture his classmates on vintage cars whether they were interested in them or not. As a result they tended to either avoid him or mimic him. Todd's teacher was concerned this was escalating and that the other children were bullying Todd, especially at break times when he was often out of sight of supervising staff. She suspected that other students were forcibly taking Todd's cars and teasing him. Todd was becoming increasingly reluctant to go out into the playground at break times and would hang back tearfully in the classroom. Todd's teacher ensured that all students, including Todd, were supervised in the playground at break times and asked staff to note any bullying.

WHAT ADDITIONAL RESOURCES CAN I ACCESS?

Financial support for students with autism varies around the world and in some countries from one region to another. Schools usually need to apply for additional resources, which are then allocated either to the school or to an individual student. A diagnosis of autism may be needed to access resources, even though it is generally accepted that resources should be allocated on the basis of needs. In some countries there is a tendency for schools and families to equate the amount of support their child receives with the number of hours they are allocated a teacher's aide. Allocating a teacher's aide or assistant is only one strategy of the many needed, as described above, that will make a school work well for students with autism. In fact, having a teacher's aide for all or part of the school day may even be counterproductive. It can make the child stand out from their peers or make them too dependent on the aide for behaviour prompts.

HOW CAN I WORK EFFECTIVELY WITH THE SCHOOL?

Try to maintain an open channel of communication with your child's school. It's great to hear when things are going well, but you also need to know when they aren't. If you hear of specific problems try to work with the school to think through strategies for modifying the environment as well as the triggers for the behaviour and its function for your child (see Chapter 5) to prevent the problem behaviour occurring. If you think there is a problem because you are worried about your child's mood or behaviour when they come home, then let the school know you are worried and work with them to find out what the problem is and to plan a solution.

Although Sue and Mike, John's parents, did a lot of planning, they did not feel the school was working with them when John started at the school. There was very little contact between the school and the family. There was a school diary which came home in John's bag every day but although Sue regularly wrote about what was happening at home and sometimes asked John's teacher questions, she found the communication from the school in the book was unreliable and often several days went by without information from school. Mike and Sue were invited to attend an individual education plan meeting after John started school but they had very little input into John's program and noted that John's teacher did not seem very interested in how much of his program was being worked on at home. At the end of Term 1, Sue and Mike arranged a meeting to discuss John's progress and explained that they were keen to be more involved. The teacher apologised for her lack of contact and focus on regular communication with them. They agreed to a weekly phone call to review the week and exchange information about John's progress and any issues arising at home and school. Sue also volunteered to come in two mornings a week to help out in the school library. Mike and Sue left feeling that Term 2 would be better.

At the same time each morning at Siew's new primary school he would become very agitated and block his ears with his hands and try to run out of the classroom. His aide tried to stop him running away by boxing him in with classroom funiture but this only increased his distress and in his desperation to escape he tried to push everything, including her, out of the way. It took Siew a long time to calm down after these incidents and it was highly disruptive for the class. His teacher and aide met with Hong Yuan and Kenneth to discuss the behaviour and Hong Yuan told them that she noticed him doing the same behaviour when they were out and there was a truck backing up making a beeping noise. His teacher realised that her classroom was next to the school canteen and every morning supplies were delivered in a truck which backed in behind the building. She now realised that Siew's outbursts were related to the sound. She asked the aide to find out when the truck made the deliveries. Hong Yuan suggested that either Siew be allowed to leave the classroom before the truck arrived and to return after it left, or they could provide him with headphones and the soundtrack of his favourite DVD and warn him when the truck was coming. They decided to try the second strategy. Because the exact delivery time varied due to traffic and the driver's other deliveries, Siew's teacher approached the truck driver and explained the situation and asked him to send her a text message when he was close to the school. He agreed, although he thought it was strange. Siew's teacher made sure she gave him feedback from time to time about the program and how well Siew was doing.

RESOURCES

Individual planning

www.positivepartnerships.com.au/planning-matrix

Visual supports

www.autismspeaks.org/docs/sciencedocs/atn/visual_supports.pdf

www.autism.org.uk/visualsupports

Emotion recognition and regulation

http://raisingchildren.net.au/articles/autism_spectrum_disorder_emotional_development.html

Apps for autism

www.learningappguide.com/AppCriteria.php

The website provides high quality, regularly updated information and critical evaluation of apps relevant to autism for an annual subscription fee.

Social and emotional skills interventions

http://onlinelibrary.wiley.com/doi/10.1002/14651858.CD008511.pub2/abstract

The Secret Agent Society: www.sst-institute.net

Social stories

www.autism.org.uk/socialstories

www.cheri.com.au/PDF_Files/professionals/Whatisasocialstory.pdf

Theory of mind interventions

http://onlinelibrary.wiley.com/doi/10.1002/14651858.CD008785.pub2/abstract

Savant skills

www.positivepartnerships.com.au/en/fact-sheet/savant-skills

Learning styles

www.positivepartnerships.com.au/learning-diversity

Bullying

www.school-portal.co.uk/GroupRenderCustomPage.asp?GroupID=891984&ResourceId=2758155

www.amaze.org.au/uploads/2011/08/Fact-Sheet-Bullying-and-Autism-Spectrum-Disorder-Aug-2011.pdf

www.autismspeaks.org/family-services/bullying

CHAPTER 8

PROBLEMS IN THE PRIMARY SCHOOL YEARS

Many problems that occur in the primary (junior) school years are not unique to this age group. Some may have been present before and persisted, or have reappeared with the changes and additional expectations that school brings. Others listed here may never occur for your child, or first appear during the secondary (high) school years. They are presented here because this is a common age for them.

ATTENTION AND CONCENTRATION

We all have different abilities to attend and concentrate and how we perform can vary depending on the setting, whether we are hungry or tired or worried, and what the task at hand is. School-aged children are no different except, as in most things, they have still not reached their full ability to pay attention and concentrate. Being able to attend and concentrate on key topics is important for learning. In the school setting more attention and concentration is expected than in the preschool and toddler years, and so any problem in this area may only come up now for the first time.

Attention and concentration can be an area of both strength and weakness in autism. One type of difficulty arises when a child has increased ability to concentrate, but that ability is limited to a special interest rather than all the important areas of learning. A child may have a high ability to concentrate on maths but is unable to shift their focus or concentrate on reading or group-based activities. In other children with autism, difficulties with attention and concentration are due to an inability to focus which limits their capacity to learn and participate.

According to *DSM-5*, children can have a diagnosis of autism spectrum disorder as well as a diagnosis of attention deficit hyperactivity disorder (ADHD). This is new to the *DSM* classification system and makes it easier to think about the types of problems your child may be experiencing (see Resources at the end of the chapter). That is, do they have both autism and ADHD, or are their attention and concentration problems primarily part of their autism? To differentiate this, increased attention and concentration on very narrowly focused interests is usually part of autism. Strategies to broaden and redirect children with high attention and concentration on a narrow topic or interest and how to use these attributes to encourage positive behaviours have been described in Chapter 6. If your child has low attention and concentration their teacher will use strategies to try to increase both in the classroom. It is best to be consistent between settings, so it is a good idea to talk to your child's teacher and find out what is being done at school, and also to share with your child's teacher any strategies that have worked well for you at home.

ATTENTION DEFICIT HYPERACTIVITY DISORDER (ADHD)

The staff at Jane's child care were concerned about her constant activity and difficulty attending to anything she was doing for more than a few minutes. They thought Jane might have attention deficit hyperactivity disorder (ADHD) and suggested to Louise that Jane be assessed at the local hospital clinic operated by a visiting paediatrician. When Jane was assessed, ADHD was considered but it was noted that Jane did not meet the criteria for a diagnosis because she was capable of sustained attention and that her behaviours were better explained by a diagnosis of autism.

Children who are diagnosed with ADHD will have problems in two key areas: (1) inattention, and (2) hyperactivity and impulsivity. The *DSM-5* criteria for a diagnosis includes descriptions like 'Often does not follow through on instructions and fails to finish schoolwork, chores, or duties in the workplace (e.g., loses focus, side-tracked)' for inattention, and 'Is often "on the go", acting as if "driven by a motor"' for hyperactivity and impulsivity.[1] For both areas, six or more criteria out of a possible nine need to be met for a diagnosis for children up to the age of sixteen and the behaviours need to have been present for at least six months (see Resources at the end of the chapter).

Behaviours seen in both key areas need to be inappropriate for a child's developmental level, not their chronological age. This is another good reason to have a clear understanding of your child's functional, cognitive and language abilities. A diagnosis of ADHD can be made in young people and adults aged seventeen or older. The criteria are slightly different and the symptoms need to have been present before the age of twelve, be present in two or more settings and to 'interfere with, or reduce the quality of, social, school, or work functioning'.[2] This is to ensure there is not an environmental trigger in one place that is leading to behaviours of the type seen in ADHD, or that the problems have just started and could be due to a specific issue like a mental illness, or a one-off trigger like a family separation. If a specific trigger or issue is identified, the management will be different. Based on the symptoms present across the key areas, different types of ADHD can be diagnosed: (1) combined presentation with both inattention and hyperactivity-impulsivity, (2) predominantly inattentive, or (3) predominantly hyperactivity-impulsivity.

Management strategies will vary with a child's age and ability and also the severity of ADHD symptoms. Evidence-based guidance is now available, with recommendations from the National Institute for Health and Care Excellence (NICE) in the UK being among the most recent (see Resources at the end of this chapter). All intervention strategies should include social, educational and psychological or behavioural interventions. For school-aged children with moderate impairment due to ADHD, the initial focus will be on parent-training programs and, for those who have an ability around the level of a typical eight-year-old, group programs that include cognitive behaviour therapy or social skills training will be recommended. These types of programs will try to improve skills, such as listening when others are talking, and provide ways for children to control themselves. If the symptoms are severe then medication may be recommended.

A child's school and teacher should be made aware of a diagnosis of ADHD and the intervention that is underway, as teaching staff are well placed to watch for any improvements or side effects and to help with behavioural management in the classroom.

The choice of medication will take into account any other problems your child has, like epilepsy or tics. There are two main drugs considered suitable for school-aged children: methylphenidate and atomoxetine. Methylphenidate is the usual first choice. Both medications act as brain stimulants and yet paradoxically improve attention and decrease aimless activity. The possible side effects of these two medications are different: commonly reported side effects for atomoxetine include nausea, dry mouth, loss of appetite, difficulty sleeping, fatigue, headache and cough; while the commonly reported side effects of methylphenidate include nervousness, either drowsiness or difficulty sleeping, and weight loss. If methylphenidate is being used, different preparations are now available that can offer slower drug release and less frequent administration.

Medication may sometimes be trialled for less severe attention and concentration problems if you and your health professional feel better attention and concentration could help with learning. This will require careful monitoring both at home and at school to ensure the goals of an improvement in attention and concentration are being met.

In some situations, another drug called clonidine may be the most appropriate medication (see also the section on sleep in Chapter 6 and the section about tics below). Clonidine has side effects, including changing blood pressure, and starting or stopping the drug needs to be closely monitored by your doctor.

SEIZURES AND EPILEPSY

Seizures are suspected when children behave in unusual ways or have 'funny turns' that seem likely to be triggered by the brain. In some instances this could be a staring episode, in others it could be a collapse to the ground with shaking or jerking. For other types of seizures it could be twitching of only one part of the body. Seizures are frightening to watch, especially if seeing one for the first time. Hopefully you will be somewhat reassured to know it is rare that a seizure causes other problems, and that most seizures stop within five minutes.

> During John's first seizure when he was ten months old his whole body jerked and he stared blankly. Sue was terrified when this happened and her first response was to call Mike. He suggested she call an ambulance. Sue's reaction to John's first seizure was only natural. It is much easier for someone who is not at the scene to think rationally.

Some behaviours or movements are typical of certain seizure types; others may indicate that seizures are likely but don't help identify the seizure type. A 'funny turn' can also be behavioural due to a movement disorder, such as a tic, or due to breathing or heart problems, especially if associated with collapse.

The two most common types of seizures in childhood are those associated with a fever (febrile seizures), usually caused by a viral illness, which affects about 5 per cent of children, or seizures after fainting. Seizures can also occur during a physical illness, or be caused by medications or ingested substances. It is best to tell your doctor about any special diet, vitamins or other complementary and alternative therapies that your child is taking, even though these are unlikely to be a cause. Seizures with a known cause usually don't need further investigation (see Resources at the end of the chapter).

Epilepsy is the diagnosis used to describe recurring seizures that are not due to fever, fainting or some other known cause. The proportion of children with autism who are diagnosed with epilepsy is similar to other children who have similar intelligence.

Epilepsy usually first occurs during the school years. There are many different types of epilepsy. The more severe kinds are usually seen early in life, often in the first weeks after birth, or during the toddler years and can cause a loss of developmental skills (see 'If skills are lost' in Chapter 3).

Many types of epilepsy in the school-aged years resolve themselves and do not require drug treatments. In deciding whether to start drug therapy, your doctor will take into account the frequency and severity of the seizures and things like whether they occur during the day and whether they could put your child's safety at risk because of possible collapse while swimming or riding a bicycle.

If your child is having a seizure you need to make sure they are in a safe place and can't fall or hurt themselves if they move. If they are on the footpath or another public place, ensure they can't hurt themselves on a hard surface and aren't in the path of cars or bikes. Do not put your finger in their mouth as this could injure them and yourself. Look at the clock. If it gets to five minutes from the onset of the seizure and your child is still fitting, call an ambulance. When possible, turn your child onto their left side and put their right arm and right leg across their body. This is known as the coma or recovery position and helps prevent a person suffocating. If your child has stopped fitting but is not responding to you, check that they are breathing and that their location is still safe. If you haven't been able to call for assistance before now, this is a good time to seek help.

If a seizure has occurred or is suspected your child may have an electroencephalogram (EEG) to assess the electrical activity of the brain. It is ideal for EEGs to be done when a child is sleep-deprived because tiredness is a known trigger for seizures. An EEG may confirm the cause of the seizure and provide more information about the location of the abnormal electrical activity. An EEG may show a pattern that is typical of epilepsy syndromes that go away after childhood, or it may show a pattern that is suggestive of a more severe problem or one that requires further investigation. In recent years, genetic and brain formation causes for epilepsy have been increasingly identified, so genetic or neuroimaging studies may also be ordered.

> After the first seizure, John had an electroencephalogram (EEG) and Mike and Sue were told he had epilepsy and needed medication. John continued to have seizures every month even when he was on medication and was seeing a medical specialist about this.

All anti-epilepsy medications, known as anticonvulsants, have side effects. Some require drug level monitoring or monitoring for side effects using blood tests. The choice of medication is based on your child's age, which medication is known to be effective for their seizure type, and any known interactions with other medications that your child is taking. Some children have severe or complex epilepsy, with more than one seizure type, and more than one medication may be needed.

As mentioned earlier, other behaviours can look like seizures. Video recordings have helped a lot with correct diagnoses. If it is not clear whether a 'funny turn' is a seizure it can be very useful to capture it on video so you can show your doctor.

MOVEMENTS YOU MIGHT NOTICE

TICS

Tics are common in all school-aged children, especially boys. They are intermittent, sudden and involuntary and can be physical movements, like grimacing or blinking, or vocalisations like throat clearing. More complicated tics are also seen — the more complicated the tic is, the more difficult it can be to distinguish it from a repetitive motor behaviour, known as a stereotypy (see next section), or an action that is voluntary and used to minimise anxiety (see Resources at the end of the chapter).

Tics are diagnosed using behavioural classification systems and the one available in *DSM-5* grades tics based on their duration, frequency and type. The three categories are: provisional tic disorder, persistent motor or vocal tic disorder, and Tourette's disorder. For a tic disorder to be diagnosed, any other possible cause of the movement or vocalisation, like medications or an underlying neurological problem, needs to have been excluded.

Most tics decrease over time. They can affect social interactions if others present are not able to ignore them and they can lead to a child being seen as different by their peers, and possibly bullied.

It is important to alert the school to your child's tics and discuss with teachers the best strategies for encouraging other children and staff to ignore them. Where tics are very frequent and causing distress to your child or having a big impact on their social or educational setting, medication may be considered. You will need to weigh up the benefits of medication against any side effects, and monitor your child's progress closely.

STEREOTYPIES

Stereotypies are also very common in young children and are also seen in older children and adults. They are repetitive motor behaviours that do not have a clear functional purpose but can be self-stimulating and include things like nail biting and thumb sucking. Doing repetitive motor behaviours is also known as 'stimming'. Behaviours commonly seen in autism, like arm flapping or head banging, are also stereotypies. To be diagnosed as a disorder, a stereotypic behaviour would have to interfere significantly with normal activities or result in self-injury.

Distinguishing a tic from a stereotypy can be difficult but in general tics are less complicated and shorter lived motor movements or sounds. It is likely that your child with autism has exhibited stereotypies at some stage. Stereotypies alone rarely justify medication, however if a behaviour is self-harming and seen in combination with other behaviours that are challenging or threatening for those caring for your child, then medication may be needed as well as a behaviour management program (see 'Managing behaviour' in Chapter 9). The types of medication used would include selective serotonin reuptake inhibitors (SSRIs) or antipsychotic medications. The choice would depend on the specific problems your child is having and, as with other medications, would be offered on a trial basis.

> When Siew started school he was still flapping his hands when he was excited or anxious, which was noticed and talked about by the other children. Siew's teacher introduced a program for the whole class about autism which explained the condition in a way the children could understand. They learnt that this funny mannerism was Siew's way of coping with things he found difficult. They also learnt about the challenges for Siew related to his autism, the things he was especially good at, and about what they could do to help him. After a while the other children stopped noticing Siew's odd behaviour and as he grew older he flapped his hands less.

OTHER MOTOR BEHAVIOURS

Some motor behaviours are driven by anxiety or a fixed and consuming interest and are known as obsessions (see 'Anxiety disorders' in Chapter 9 for more on obsessive compulsive disorder). Differentiating behaviours of this type from tics and motor stereotypies is not easy. If a motor behaviour, such as picking at skin, is triggered by anxiety or linked to an obsession, then not being allowed to enact it will increase the child's level of anxiety and show up as distress. In this way, although the behaviour has no specific motor purpose, it fulfils an important psychological need. Verbal children can explain when they feel stress and tension or have an obsessional thought that is relieved by a motor action, but only when they reach a sufficient age or ability. This means you and the professionals you are working with are often left guessing about whether there are specific triggers to the behaviours you see. To complicate things further, both tics and stereotypies can increase when children are in stressful situations or are anxious for known reasons. The reason for the increase in tics and stereotypies in these types of situations is not well understood. As such, the treatment of motor behaviours, as described above, is usually based on whether the behaviour itself is interrupting important activities or causing harm. If intervention is needed, then the same medications used for severe stereotypies are usually prescribed on a trial basis (see Resources at the end of the chapter).

ABSCONDING

In autism, absconding is usually not a wilful act but the result of a child moving towards an interest or away from a situation that they find stressful or threatening. Absconding can put your child's safety at risk and, like other unwanted behaviours, it is important to understand the reasons driving the behaviour and to address any issues that can be changed. Anyone who is involved in caring for your child in a setting where they abscond needs to be engaged as they may have observed important events prior to your child leaving and will also need to be part of any changes that are made to prevent absconding.

In some situations it is possible and necessary to modify the environment to minimise the risk of your child leaving. Child-proof locks or latches that are too high to reach can work well during the younger years. Furniture should not be able to be moved near to windows, fences, gates or to allow better access to safety locks. If your child is known to leave during the night when unattended, then alarm systems on doors and windows may be necessary.

Being prepared can also help. Introduce your child to police officers so they can see that police are safe and helpful adults. Take a photograph of your child if you are going to a crowded place so you will be able to accurately describe their appearance and clothing if you are separated from them. If your child is a frequent absconder you can also notify your neighbours so they will let you know if they see your child on the street or climbing a fence. You can also let your local police know about your child's interests and likely places he or she could go. Although tracking devices are used by some families and have been found to work well, they are not enough on their own, as they can either fail to work or be removed (see Resources at the end of the chapter).

PUBERTY

Towards the end of the primary school years your child will enter puberty. Most young people with autism experience the physical changes of puberty in the same way as other young people. What can be more complex is developing an understanding of the physical changes that have occurred, the associated sexual feelings they are experiencing and the social understanding of what, where and when sexual behaviours are acceptable.

Advice about dealing with puberty is very similar to advice for other aspects of change and behaviour management for children and young people with autism (see 'Managing behaviour' in Chapter 9). The most important thing is to make sure your child is adequately prepared for this important change. If you have a girl then specific information about preparation for periods is also needed. If you have concerns about any of the physical changes your young person with autism is experiencing, you should consult your local doctor for advice. For girls, changes in mood or behaviour may occur before their periods. If these changes are causing problems, then effective treatments are available. Menstrual irregularity, heavy bleeding or severe pain with menstruation can also be managed with physical therapies like heat and massage for pain relief. It is worth seeking medical advice if these problems persist or do not respond well to the usual remedies.

> Jane became increasingly anxious before each period which was accompanied by agitation and refusal to leave the house and locking herself in her room. She had lots of trouble with cramps. Louise would massage her lower back and give her a hot water bottle. Louise let Jane stay home from school at these times, especially when Jane was particularly anxious and irritable.

Personal hygiene is important and needs to be attended to by your young person or someone who is caring for them. Again, the usual principles of behaviour change apply here, so start early, ideally before any physical changes have started, and address any specific issues that could occur because of your child's sensory problems, and provide information in a format, such as a schedule, that is at the right level of your child's understanding (see Resources at the end of the chapter).

ANXIETY

> For Todd, anxiety was a major challenge during the school years. When he first started school he insisted that in any room he was in all the cupboard doors had to be closed and all the tissues had to be tucked into their boxes. This improved but his teachers noticed it would recur when it was time for a public speaking

session. His parents found a child psychologist who was experienced in anxiety management and had also worked with children with autism. She assessed Todd and recommended cognitive behaviour therapy. His parents reviewed information about cognitive behaviour therapy for anxiety in general and for children with autism and talked further with the psychologist about how she would do this with Todd. They decided that an approach that helped Todd think about why he was tucking tissues into boxes and closing doors, to discuss his fears of public speaking and to work with him to manage those behaviours might be effective. They decided to monitor Todd's door-closing and tissue-tucking behaviour at school, with the help of his teachers, to assess whether the intervention was working. Not long after the six sessions ended Todd was able to sit through a public speaking session and give his talk without closing cupboard doors or tucking tissues. His parents asked his teachers to continue to monitor this behaviour for three months after the intervention and were pleased that there had been other sessions that had gone well. Because Todd was still anxious in situations where unexpected changes occurred, they decided to visit the psychologist again to ask whether this too might respond to cognitive behaviour therapy.

Anxiety in the primary school years has much in common with anxiety at any other age. For strategies to deal with this, see Chapter 9. Anxiety may also be due to bullying at any age. See the sections on bullying in chapters 7 and 9 for further discussion and strategies.

PREPARING FOR SECONDARY SCHOOL

The move from primary school to secondary school is a major step for most children.

> For John the transition to secondary school was not necessary because the school he attended continued for the secondary school years. The processes and supports he had in place in primary school continued consistently through his secondary school years to encourage him to learn, communicate and increase wanted behaviours. In secondary school, the focus of John's program shifted to increasing his independence and developing vocational skills.

If your young person is enrolled in a regular primary school, either in a special class for children with learning difficulties or a regular class with or without specialist support, they are most likely to continue their education in a regular secondary school. The transition will be smoother if they are able to stay at the same school, however, in most cases, moving to secondary school means a different school in a different location. Secondary school brings a change in both academic and social expectations. The professionals you know well will help and the same steps employed during the transition to primary school (see Chapter 7) can be helpful, if adjusted to suit your child's abilities and difficulties and their change in maturity. Again, preparation is essential both for your child and for the receiving school. Ideally, the school will ask for information about your child, their strengths and needs and the sorts of adjustments and accommodations that are in place and working well in the primary school setting. For example, if your child has access to a sanctuary space at primary school and this is helping them to manage anxiety and distress related to sensory overload in the crowded playground, then they will need the same in secondary school.

For your child, a series of visits to their new school in the final term of their primary school year plus visual supports, like photos of their new school and new teachers, which they can review with you, will help them prepare for the change. Additional strategies that could help in secondary school include visually coded timetables with colours for different subjects plus possible coloured dots on the relevant books and equipment matching these subjects, as organisational demands will be higher. This could help them to get to classes with the right gear. The better prepared the school and the student, the smoother the transition is likely to be.

> Jessica, Todd's mum, was very worried about the transition to secondary school because she now knew all the staff at his primary school and knew how much they kept on eye on Todd and made sure he was coping in the classroom and the playground. Some of the children in Todd's class were going to the local secondary school but after careful consideration Jessica and Joseph decided that Todd would be more likely to get the support he needed at a secondary school run by the same religious organisation as his primary school, despite the fact that it was not as close to home and meant Jessica would have to continue to drive Todd to and from school each day. One of the reasons for this decision was that the principal at the secondary school had experience with young people with autism. Several students with autism were enrolled in the school and some of the teaching staff and the deputy principal had attended a training program designed to enable the school to develop individual programs for these students. Jessica had heard that the staff adapted the academic curriculum to suit students with autism and the school made changes to the environment and systems that would make it possible for the students with autism to cope. For example, the school had an

allocated room in the library supervised by library staff where the students could go at break times away from the noise and social demands of the playgrounds. There were also weekly groups where the students could share their special interests.

RESOURCES

Attention deficit hyperactivity disorder (*DSM-5* criteria)

www.cdc.gov/ncbddd/adhd/diagnosis.html

Guidelines for ADHD

www.nice.org.uk/guidance/cg72/chapter/guidance#treatment-for-children-and-young-people

Seizure facts and action plan

www.rch.org.au/kidsinfo/fact_sheets/Seizures_safety_issues_and_how_to_help

Tics (DSM-5 diagnostic criteria)

www.cdc.gov/ncbddd/tourette/diagnosis.html

Stimming (stereotypies)

http://raisingchildren.net.au/articles/autism_spectrum_disorder_stimming.html

Informing the students in the school about autism

http://fhautism.com/the-sixth-sense-ii-sharing-information-about-autism-spectrum-disorders-with-general-education-students.html#.VFfgfCjcJUQ

There is a small cost for this program.

Special interests and restricted repetitive behaviours

www.autism.org.uk/living-with-autism/understanding-behaviour/obsessions-repetitive-behaviours-and-routines.aspx

Absconding

www.autismireland.ie/assets/files/JenDocs/IAApreventingabsconding.pdf

Puberty and general hygiene

> http://raisingchildren.net.au/articles/autism_spectrum_disorder_
> puberty_teenagers.html/context/886

> http://raisingchildren.net.au/articles/autism_spectrum_disorder_
> personal_hygiene_teenagers.html

> www.amaze.org.au/uploads/2011/08/Fact-Sheet-Puberty-and-Autism-
> Spectrum-Disorders-Aug-2011.pdf

Preparing for menstruation (periods) and managing premenstrual symptoms

> http://raisingchildren.net.au/articles/autism_spectrum_disorder_
> periods.html

CHAPTER 9

THE SECONDARY SCHOOL YEARS

While much of this book has dealt with specific issues and problems that can arise for children with autism, it's important to remember that watching a young person with autism negotiate the many challenges of life can be extraordinarily rewarding and often fill you with pride. As young people with autism develop an understanding of the world around them, they offer many insights into their own unique perspective and a refreshingly different view of the world. They grow to understand their own behaviours and develop some understanding of the behaviours of others. They notice things a typical young person either may not have thought of or may not have shared with you. Young people with autism can also have some extraordinary skills and abilities. As they get older, opportunities increase for these to be further developed and shared with others.

Young people entering secondary (high) school are going through a stage of rapid growth in their knowledge, self-management, autonomy and emotion regulation. During these years typical young people look more towards peers and other adults as role models, and less towards their parents and other carers.

There is emerging evidence that the brains of young people are changing in important ways that, even for those who have been able to communicate effectively previously, mean they become less able to listen to others and more self-concerned. Although during the secondary school years young people are being given more opportunities to manage themselves, in many young people the frontal lobes of their brains are not fully developed, so they have less feedback to monitor their behaviour compared with older adults. This is thought to be the reason for much of the risk-taking behaviour seen during the secondary school and early adult years. Emotional understanding increases in complexity and with that comes changes in patterns of mood for some young people. An understanding of what is right and wrong becomes contextualised and more complex. At the same time, physical changes mean rapid growth and gains in strength. Sexual maturation is occurring physically, as is an understanding of gender and sexual identity. The underlying factors influencing the changes that create the typical patterns of behaviours associated with young people are not fully understood, but sex hormones, like testosterone and oestrogen, are implicated for obvious reasons. Also during the secondary school years, young people develop a better understanding of their place in society, and they realise that they and those they care for are not invincible.

Your young person with autism will be experiencing all this and may face additional challenges because of the way they interact, organise themselves and learn, and also because their interests may not be the same as other young people their age. They may appear to be immune from peer pressure because of their lack of interest in current fads and trends, that is, what is cool and what is not. They may, in fact, find the behaviour of their peers pretty bizarre. Your young person with autism can be supported to better manage both the academic aspects of secondary school as well as the social aspects, also called the 'hidden curriculum' (see below for more discussion and Resources at the end of the chapter) so they can participate in school and learn the social and academic skills they need to enable them to fully participate in society in whatever way is best for them.

CHOOSING A SCHOOL

By now you will have experience with the education system. The types of placement available for secondary school will be similar to those available for the primary (junior school) years (see Chapter 7). The questions to ask of your child's prospective secondary school are similar to those you asked when your child was starting primary school. Depending on where you live there will be more or less choice. Finding the best fit for your child depends on their strengths and needs, what works for them, and the options available. For some children, a regular secondary school with some support may work well. For others, especially those with significant intellectual impairment, a special school or a special unit in a regular school may be the best option. Like primary schools, special secondary schools or units may be autism-specific or cater for a range of young people with special needs. It is likely that you will be working closely with staff from the education system your child is enrolled in at primary school to identify options and facilitate the transition to secondary school (see Resources at the end of the chapter).

In special schools and units, secondary school will be similar to primary school with the focus on individual programs, small classes and consistent staffing. Program content should be appropriate to your child's age and stage of development and, like primary school, is likely to involve some form of the mainstream curriculum adapted and adjusted to your child's strengths and needs, as well as goals to target their individual characteristics. The focus should be on learning to be independent and working towards the development of vocational skills with supported transition to post-school options and ideally further study, training or employment.

> Siew went to the local secondary school but he struggled academically and socially. He had some subject areas in which he was stronger than others, like science and computing, but he was behind the class even in these.

He also had great difficulty understanding language that dealt with human thoughts and feelings and failed to understand the rules and regulations that governed the social interactions of his peers and the adults around him. He had trouble getting himself to his classes at the right time with the right equipment and books and never knew what he was supposed to do for homework. Siew became increasingly anxious in his first year of secondary school, his hand flapping escalated and he started hitting his head with his fists. Hong Yuan and Kenneth decided to move so they could enrol him in another school some distance away where there was a specialised unit for students with autism. Hong Yuan had a friend from the parent support group whose son was also enrolled there. Siew began his second year of secondary school in the specialised unit in a small group of eight students with staff who understood the supports he needed to cope with both the academic and the social side of school life. They focused on providing predictable routines, ensuring that Siew and his classmates understood what was expected of them and that the boys were able to communicate. Siew's anxiety reduced as did his odd mannerisims and head-hitting behaviour.

WHAT'S DIFFERENT IN SECONDARY SCHOOL

For young people with autism who attend a regular secondary school the differences between primary and secondary school are marked. Secondary school students are expected to be more independent and cope with a complex timetable and different teachers and rooms for different subjects. There is likely to be more pressure academically, both in terms of the curriculum and how your child will be expected to work. Academically, students with autism have areas of strength and weakness. There will be classes where your young person will struggle and classes where they will do well. In terms of the processes in secondary school, there may be issues arising from difficulties with planning and organisation, managing time and understanding 'the big picture' or broader context. You may find your young person is struggling because there is less structure, particularly during free periods which now occur more often.

All students have to deal with what is sometimes described as the 'hidden curriculum'. This refers to unspoken cultural and social information and rules governing the social aspects of school life and adolescence. The hidden curriculum dictates how students should interact with peers, teachers and other adults and what ideas and behaviours are considered acceptable or unacceptable. This is rarely spelt out and most young people understand it without needing to be taught. This may not be the case for a young person with autism, who may have difficulty because of their limited understanding of communication nuances and imagining what might be in the minds of others (see Resources at the end of the chapter).

Your young person may appear emotionally or socially immature and naïve because they have a limited understanding of the nature and range of their own and other people's emotions, and the triggers for the emotionally based behaviours around them. They may show a lack of interest in peers, typical adolescent social activities and the latest trends. They may be direct, literal and truthful. A literal understanding of right and wrong, that may have helped your child traverse the primary school years, is now likely to be seen as rigid. A tendency to take things literally and a lack of insight into the motivations of others may also result in your young person with autism becoming involved in dangerous or even illegal activities. It is best to talk about these risks with your young person, in a similar way to discussing drug and alcohol use (more on this below). If feelings of distress and confusion, created by the new pressures of their complex social environment, are unrecognised, they can lead to mood or behaviour problems, which may only be noticed as behavioural change (more on this below too).

Transition into secondary school needs to be carefully planned. Jane had a disasterous experience in her first year of high school and ended up at home on a distance education program. A new principal at the school changed that when he set up a transition program for her.

> Before school started Louise went to a meeting with the principal, a specialist support teacher from the regional office and some of the staff who would be teaching Jane. Together they discussed Jane's strengths and challenges, decided what was most important to work on and developed a plan to support Jane to return to school. The plan included a transition program to prepare Jane for school with photos and stories about what was going to happen, who she would meet, and what she should do and say. Jane also had a schedule gradually increasing the amount of time she spent at school so she understood what was going to happen each day and to prompt Louise and her teachers to explain any changes to her. One teacher agreed to be the primary support person for Jane and to ensure all staff were aware of her program. The school agreed to help Jane understand her own emotions, and how to calm herself when she was angry. A special space was set aside for Jane to go to when things were getting too much for her and she had a card she carried with her to show staff when she needed a break. Louise agreed to help with the emotion understanding and management program at home too. Academically, the school provided a specially adapted curriculum for Jane which included task sheets to break down activities into small manageable steps. Jane's program started a few weeks before the beginning of the first term and involved visits to the school and opportunities for Jane to meet staff who would be her teachers, especially

her mentor. Jane started school initially staying until morning break, then increasing the time she spent at school until she attended full time. Her teaching team met regularly with Louise and began to include Jane in meetings as well to review the program and make any adjustments when needed.

In her book, *Martian in the Playground*, Clare Sainsbury describes what it is like to be at school for a child with autism: 'I don't understand the children around me. They frighten and confuse me ... I try so hard to do what I am told, but just when I think I am being most helpful and good, the teachers tell me off and I don't know why. It's as if everybody is playing some complicated game and I am the only one who hasn't been told the rules.'[1]

As a result, managing the social side of secondary-school life can be more challenging than dealing with the academic curriculum.

> Todd had more difficulty at school getting on in the playground than he did in class with his studies. He didn't share any interests with the other boys in his year and his language and conversation tended to be very formal and pedantic. He did, however, tell Jessica that he would like to have friends, although she wondered if he really understood much about friendship. Jessica spoke to the teacher who mentored Todd. They found a local car club where vintage car enthusiasts met and worked on restoring old cars. Even though Todd was too young to drive, they approached the club about allowing him to join to work on car restoration on Saturday mornings. Todd had always found it easier to relate to adults than peers. At school his teacher arranged for Todd to spend break times in the library where he could research his favourite topics. He felt less need to have friends at school once he joined the car club and met like-minded people there each week.

This means that it is important to work with the school to ensure your young person's considerable strengths and abilities are appreciated and they have the support they need, especially outside the classroom.

AUTISM RULES, OK!

Listening to your young person with autism is extremely important. You need to do this and reinforce what they are saying with the school. The goals your young person is working on need to be goals they value. They should have input into the planning and review process to ensure they have some ownership of the goals, otherwise chances of success are slim. The aim is not to make them 'normal', whatever that may be. Your young person is unique and their autism is part of that uniqueness and who they are. Valuing and embracing that is important, and the school should do the same. This is increasingly relevant in adolescence and is essential to minimise mental health problems that may result from the stress and anxiety of not being understood, not understanding what is going on in the social world, being perceived negatively and not coping (see section below for more on mental health problems).

The school should support your young person to participate, but schools vary in the extent to which they are able and willing to do this. People with autism are historically not good self-advocates. While there are now more autistic voices being heard, at an individual level for your young person with autism it is still likely to be difficult. So try to find a way to hear about their experiences, challenges and aspirations. They are likely to have reduced or patchy insight into their own behaviour and will need support to come up with strategies to recognise and manage their own emotional response and recognise emotional responses in others. You can help a lot by encouraging your young person to speak for themselves, while continuing to be their co-advocate or to heavily support their self-advocacy.

WHAT MAKES SCHOOL WORK

The characteristics of successful secondary schools are the same as the characteristics of successful primary schools (see Chapter 7). Positive teacher attributes are just as important, although in regular secondary school your young person with autism will have several teachers and it probably isn't reasonable to expect them to all have high levels of experience and expertise in working with students with autism. What is recommended is that there is one staff member in the school who knows your young person well, has expertise in autism and the capacity to be a case manager or mentor. This person can advocate for your child with other staff and may also be responsible for the individual educational planning process. In addition, it is important your young person's teachers know about relevant parts of their individual program and the goals and strategies being used to help them. Ensuring that this process is in place and the whole school community is engaged is the role of the school principal. Good leadership is critically important in secondary schools.

INDIVIDUAL PLANNING

As in primary school, individual planning is an important component of your young person's education. Every young person with autism has a unique combination of strengths and needs and each school has specific characteristics that need to be taken into account. The development of the plan is likely to be facilitated by a special education staff member, who may be based at the school or may work with several schools. The program should include consideration of the adaptations and accommodations your young person needs to manage the curriculum and the strategies needed to address issues arising from their characteristics, especially the development of social skills. It is important to keep in mind the difference between learning social skills and being sociable. Your child will need to learn specific skills in social situations to get by, even if they never find social interaction in itself rewarding or enjoyable. The general principles for good individual planning in secondary school are the same as for primary school (see Chapter 7).

> Students with autism in Todd's school also had support from a specialist itinerant teacher employed to work across several schools and provide expert advice about the best way to adapt education programs and the school environment for these students. Unfortunately, not all the teachers at Todd's school were supportive of the specialised program for the students with autism and some refused to make any concessions in their teaching. For example, one teacher continued to tell the class about their homework assignments without providing the information in writing, which meant Todd never knew what homework he was expected to do for this class and got into trouble as a result.

SUPPORTS

For some young people with autism, a lack of interest in their peers is protective. During a time that is often marked by turmoil and increased complexity of relationships, they simply avoid situations that create these sorts of dilemmas. However, if your young person with autism is keen to make friends, this can be a particularly difficult time. Conforming is more important during adolescence and the nuances of social interactions increase in complexity in secondary school. Peer groups may be defined by subtle non-verbal communication patterns or styles of clothing, while emotional and increasingly intimate connections are coming to the fore. It can also be a time when problems that were not as obvious become more easily noticed. It is important to ensure that your young person's peers have an understanding of autism and how it affects your child. Proactive strategies, such as setting up lunchtime special interest groups and nominating peer buddies, may also help.

Many strategies exist to assist young people in secondary school. Some of the practical academic supports include homework assistance, provision of a laptop or scribe (note taker) or extra time for exams, and offering an adapted academic curriculum perhaps with a reduced number of subjects. Some of the ways to manage the school environment include provision of a sanctuary space, while others include allowing flexibility for the school uniform, attendance at assemblies and sporting activities, and offering support for special interests. Secondary schools should provide transition support to your young person's next setting.

> In the final years of secondary school Jane completed a specially adapted curriculum which gave her an additional year to complete her senior schooling and reduced the number of subjects completed each semester or term, which decreased her anxiety. As she approached school-leaving age, staff at the school worked with Louise to find a place at a tertiary college where she could continue to develop her information technology skills.

BULLYING

All aspects of the discussion about bullying in the primary school section (see Chapter 7) also apply in secondary school. In secondary school, bullying may increase and can be more sophisticated and subtle. It may include social exclusion or isolation, spreading lies and false rumours, having money or other things taken or damaged, being threatened or being forced to do things. Sexual bullying and cyber bullying, via phone, email or social media, also occur. Many teenagers with autism say that they find the small talk of other teenagers tedious and alien, and they don't find social interaction a relaxing or enjoyable experience. While some young people with autism are not bothered by social isolation, for others who are keen to be involved with peers and to be like them, social isolation can have a big impact. You may not hear about bullying even if you ask about it directly. You may instead notice changes of behaviour, mood and school performance. Any of the mental health problems discussed below could be the first clue that bullying is taking place. Given that the secondary school years are ones in which mental health problems often first appear, it is important to consider bullying as a possible cause of any change in your young person (see Resources at the end of the chapter).

Strategies to manage bullying should focus on prevention. Examples in secondary schools include providing a dedicated quiet area for students, that students who do not have autism may also use. The development of social skills should be an important part of the curriculum but needs to be carefully planned, structured and delivered. We can teach young people with autism the social behaviours they need but we can't teach them to be sociable. Learning about social interaction is unlikely to be achieved by forcing students to spend their 'down time' in noisy, overwhelming environments. Some schools have had great success with lunch clubs. These are supervised by staff and provide structured activities during longer break times. Any student can join a club, and activities are chosen by the students according to their interests.

Bullying is less likely to occur if your young person is in the company of a supportive group. Introducing mentors or mentor groups is a more age-appropriate strategy than the 'circle of friends' suggested for primary-school settings. The mentor or mentor group look out for your young person or support them during identified risk times. It is important to ensure that the mentors have a clear understanding of their responsibilities and of the difficulties the young person with autism faces, and are themselves supported by all staff.

Every school will have a policy and procedures for dealing with bullying. Both your child and their peers will need to be involved in working toward a solution if bullying occurs, as they were with Todd.

> While the school provided a range of supports in the
> classroom and grounds, unfortunately there were some

students who bullied Todd, copying his unusual voice and way of talking. They tried to get him on his own away from staff and other students and pushed him around when they could. At school they forced him to give them his vintage cars and threw them over the school fence. When Todd retaliated by hitting out at them they reported him to the teacher supervising the playground. Fortunately, the teacher realised there was likely to be a reason for Todd's unusual aggression towards the other students and took the time to sit down with Todd and talk to him calmly to find out what was happening. Staff then found several students who were willing to become Todd's mentors to keep an eye out for him. They also organised an information session about autism for these students and included the bullies to ensure that both the bullies and the buddies understood the strengths and difficulties of their peers with autism.

In some ways now it is cool to be a geek and positive representation of this in the media is growing. This type of social change will also be helpful in preventing bullying.

SEXUALITY AND RELATIONSHIPS

Sexuality develops in the person with autism the same as for other young people. One difference is that young people who do not have autism build on their understanding about sexuality and sexual relationships with information they gather from their peers, social media and watching others. In a young person with autism, some of this information may need to be presented in a more direct and adult-led way.

Understanding personal boundaries and how there are differences in physical closeness for family, close friends and others may need to be specifically taught. Providing information about this in advance may prevent problems later.

Masturbation can cause problems if overused as a way of relieving tension or if used in inappropriate settings. An understanding of sexual function and its link to emotional and physical intimacy is important. Education about private versus public places is also important and should be taught in anticipation of the onset of puberty and the development of sexuality.

You may also be concerned that your young person with autism may not know the difference between a healthy and unhealthy relationship and acceptable versus unacceptable touching. Discussing this before emotional and physical relationships develop is ideal (see Resources at the end of the chapter).

MANAGING BEHAVIOUR

Teenage years may bring additional behaviour challenges. Disruptive behaviours may appear for the first time or evolve into behaviours that are more challenging to manage because of your child's increased size and strength. This was the case for Siew when his head banging escalated at his first secondary school. Principles of behaviour management are the same as those described in Chapter 5. A couple of things are different. Having autism, which is not a physically obvious disability, at an age when behaviour problems are more common generally, can sometimes lead teachers and peers to judge behaviour as simply obstructive or difficult, without trying to understand the reason for it. Also, with growth and increased strength, behaviours that might not have been as problematic earlier on may become more disruptive or potentially dangerous for the young person with autism or for others. For example, a young child who drops to the ground and refuses to budge when Mum tries to take him into the shopping mall is not so unusual. As a last resort Mum can pick him up and take him to the car, but the same behaviour becomes very noticable and unusual in a young person in their teens, and they are now too strong and heavy for Mum to move. Finding out the trigger and function of the behaviour is essential, as covered previously. Remember, adolescence can be a difficult time for all young people and those with autism are no exception (see Resources at the end of the chapter).

AGGRESSIVE BEHAVIOURS

The goal should always be to have programs and strategies in place to prevent aggressive behaviour (both verbal and physical) occurring. There are usually signs that a young person with autism is building up to a behavioural outburst, which as a parent you will recognise. You will also know what the usual triggers are for such an outburst, like changes in routine or interference with a ritual. Knowing if there are any underlying thoughts or emotional problems is important. The goal is always to prevent challenging behaviour occurring in the first place with a program that includes teaching your young person to recognise things that upset or stress them and their reactions to triggers, and what to do when they start to feel agitated. This could be calm breathing, asking for a break or moving away from other people.

Aggression towards other students may also occur at school and is likely to be related to something other students are doing. The school needs to become involved here in the same way as for bullying.

The best way to manage challenging behaviour is to be well prepared. If this has been an ongoing problem then both a long-term behaviour management plan and a short-term crisis management plan need to be developed. All staff working with your child should be informed and understand what to do in the event of a crisis.

Aggressive behaviour can still occur. The most important thing is to try to stay calm and do what you can to make your young person and those around them safe. If possible, move people away and direct your young person to a calm, quiet place to give them the chance to recover. Keep speech to a minimum. Even young people with good language skills will be overwhelmed by too much talking when they are very stressed. Restraint should be used only as a last resort to keep people safe. In this situation you will need to inform people your child has autism and you may need to get help from emergency services.

Medication is only used when behavioural approaches have failed, either in a crisis situation or as a non-crisis intervention. Either way, it should always be used in conjunction with behavioural management as one part of a strategy to ensure safety for your young person with autism and for others. In a crisis situation either a minor tranquiliser (such as a benzodiazepine) or an atypical antipsychotic agent will be used, while for longer term use an atypical antipsychotic is likely to be used (see Resources at the end of the chapter).

SELF-INJURING BEHAVIOUR

The reasons for self-injuring or self-harming behaviour can be complex. In autism, a young person could be injuring themselves as part of a repetitive behaviour and the injury is secondary but not intentional. They may be injuring themselves through frustration, perhaps because of communication difficulties. In other instances, self-injury could occur as a short-term way of coping with unpleasant feelings and thoughts. Young people with autism will be experiencing a range of stressful events, which they may not be able to share with others. Uncommon but important causes of self-injuring behaviour include psychotic or suicidal thoughts. For example, if a young person with autism believed that small aliens were living under their skin this might result in a picking behaviour (for more information, see the section about psychoses below). Suicidal thoughts should trigger urgent medical assessment even if self-injuring actions would not be enough to end life. It is the severity of the depression and the intent that requires immediate psychiatric input (for more information, see the section about depression below).

The first step is to check whether there are any physical problems present (see Chapter 5). A long-standing relationship with your doctor can help in this situation as they will know whether the behaviour is different to a usual pattern and will be able to assess if harm is being caused by the behaviour over time.

The primary goal of intervention is to prevent injury and some simple strategies may achieve this, such as ensuring a place of safety, and removing dangerous items. For a longer term solution it is important to identify if the behaviour serves a function or if it is the manifestation of one of the problems described above. If the triggers and function of self-injuring behaviour are not apparent and a simple solution does not assist, you should seek expert advice.

John's teacher noted that John had characteristic sensory seeking behaviours and that when he was stressed and agitated he sometimes would injure himself. He was constantly on the move around the classroom. Even when sitting on a chair, he rocked backwards and forwards in it or swung back onto the chair's back legs. She noted he often did things like spinning around on the spot, jumping up and down, flapping his hands and fingers, and making high-pitched squealing noises while at the same time covering his ears. She understood he was having difficulty self-regulating his arousal levels and could quickly and very easily become agitated. At these times when he was very stressed, his teacher noted John was likely to injure himself by biting his fingers and hitting his face with his hands. She made careful observations about the times and situations these behaviours occurred and discussed the situation with Mike and Sue. John's self-injuring behaviour increased when he was in a crowded noisy environment, when first arriving at school and when there was an unexpected change in routine. His teacher arranged with Sue to meet John at a side gate to the school first thing in the morning to avoid the noise and bustle of the other students arriving and together they worked on providing John with visual supports to manage changes in routine and to gradually increase his tolerance. After six months John's self-injuring behaviour only occurred rarely.

MENTAL HEALTH PROBLEMS

Mental health problems are common in the secondary school years and more common in young people with autism. The reported frequency depends on what is included as a mental health problem, but most studies report that most young people with autism will experience a mental health problem at some point, with anxiety problems the most common. Many of the more serious problems described below are infrequent and won't be an issue for your child, but they are worth knowing about so you can take appropriate action early if they do arise.

ANXIETY DISORDERS

There are several different anxiety disorders. As discussed in chapters 5 and 7, anxiety is a common problem for children with autism and the same is true for young people.

If an anxiety disorder is creating panic symptoms or leads to a panic attack, it can seem like a medical emergency but this is not the case. Panic attacks can bring on physiological manifestations such as finding it hard to catch your breath, a racing heart, trembling or shaking, and sweatiness. The person having the panic attack can feel very scared and may think they are going to die. A panic attack may often look like a serious medical problem and it is not uncommon for individuals having their first panic attack to visit an emergency department. An important part of treating an acute panic attack is to understand that it is not a medical emergency, and to offer reassurance and comfort.

As well as the usual strategies for managing behaviour, like identifying known triggers, some more specific interventions can work. Any stimulants, like smoking or drinking energy drinks containing caffeine, should be stopped. Relaxation activities can also be helpful. The trigger may be something that affects all young people, like worrying about failing at school, or an autism-related problem, like difficulties with social interaction. Learning to recognise signs of emotion in yourself and in others is very important and is something that young people with autism often have to learn. There are several useful programs for older and younger children with autism to help with this that we refer to in Chapter 7. Once young people with autism learn to recognise signs of emotional arousal, they can learn strategies to help them regulate these emotions.

There are also effective interventions for anxiety based on cognitive behaviour therapy, which can be used for young people with a mental age of eight or more. Cognitive behaviour therapy can be effective for both identifying triggers, if there are any, and creating coping strategies, as described for Todd in Chapter 8. There are also effective drug therapies for anxiety that can be tried if other management is insufficient. It is important to work with the professionals involved to monitor progress in order to decide whether to continue or stop a therapy, to monitor side effects and to determine if alternatives are needed. For detailed information to assist with a step-wise approach to best management see guidelines provided by the National Institute of Clinical Excellence (NICE) listed in Resources at the end of the chapter.

Jane's first weeks at secondary school did not go smoothly and she became increasingly anxious and distressed. Louise started letting her stay at home and made an appointment for her to see the local child and youth mental health service where she was prescribed medication to reduce her anxiety. She returned to school with her mother driving her there and back for a while and seemed to be coping, although Jade (Jane's sister) reported that Jane spent break times in the classroom by herself and didn't mix with the other students in the playground at all. Jane was assigned a teacher's aide (assistant) for two hours a day to help her, however the aide was not trained in autism and worked with Jane in class not at break times. Louise found she was being rung two to three times a week and asked to come and collect Jane because of outbursts at school. At these times Louise found Jane very distressed and unable to tell her about what had happened. Staff told Louise that Jane had 'meltdowns' where she had been aggressive towards them or to her peers. After a few weeks Louise gave up coaxing Jane into the car to go to school and decided to keep her at home. She continued the medication but wasn't convinced it was helping. Jane was home-schooled for the rest of her first secondary school year. Louise received some support from the distance education unit.

When the principal at Jane's school changed, so did the approach to her education. Staff recognised that there were triggers, things that made Jane feel anxious, that came before her aggressive behaviour. School staff developed a behaviour support plan designed to prevent outbursts occurring. Jane also took part in a life skills program with a focus on developing skills to manage reactions to change of circumstances, improving functional communication skills, implementing strategies to manage triggers and understanding the appropriate behaviours and skills to survive in society, such as purchasing items, accessing services such as libraries, and taking transport. As her challenging behaviour settled, Jane and her mother returned to the youth mental health service and developed a plan for a gradual reduction of her anti-anxiety medication.

As Jane grew and matured she learnt to manage her anxiety better by avoiding known triggers and practising calming strategies when she felt herself becoming anxious.

Obsessive compulsive disorder (OCD) is a particular type of anxiety disorder. A person with OCD experiences thoughts that make them act in a certain way, which then reduces their anxiety. If they are unable to act in the way they want, their anxiety will increase. OCD is hard to diagnose if a young person is not able to describe why they are acting in the way that is seen, and is therefore difficult to distinguish from repetitive behaviours that may be part of autism. The treatment for OCD involves psychological therapies but a different type to that used for other anxiety disorders. Similar medications can also be effective, and monitoring is again needed.

DEPRESSION

Depression is an extreme form of sadness that interferes with life. Young people with autism may find it harder than others their age to describe how they feel and so their behaviour is an important indicator that they may be depressed. If depression is severe it can lead to inactivity, poor sleep, little interest in things that are usually of interest, and loss of appetite. In the most severe episodes a young person could think that the way they feel is intolerable and have suicidal thoughts. Thinking that is out of touch with reality, also known as psychotic thinking (see section below), can occur in severe depression. This can lead a young person to harm themselves or others. If a young person has suicidal or psychotic thoughts seek medical help immediately.

People can become depressed if they are unhappy with their circumstances or because of sad or stressful events, like the death of a loved one or parents separating. In autism it can occur as a young person develops an understanding of the way they are. Management of depression will depend on the triggers, severity and the risks identified. As for anxiety, psychological therapy alone or in combination with medication is known to be effective, but requires monitoring and varying levels of supervision.

PSYCHOSES

There are different types of psychotic episodes and there are also disorders associated with psychosis, of which schizophrenia is probably the best known. Psychotic disorders can co-occur with depression and can drive self-injuring behaviours. They can be caused by prescribed or non-prescribed drugs. Some psychotic episodes occur only once while others recur (see Resources at the end of the chapter).

Young people with autism are three times more likely to have a psychotic episode than their peers, but the prevalence is still low, at around 3 per cent. Why there are increased rates of psychoses in young adults with autism is not yet fully explained, with emerging findings of some shared genetic risk. It is likely that there will be different pathways for different individuals with autism.

Psychosis in autism can also be hard to identify and may only be picked up through changes in behaviour. If you are concerned about a particular behaviour change, it is best to seek advice from a medical professional. Medication will be needed to manage psychosis, along with other measures. Unfortunately, the evidence for positive effects of antipsychotic medication in young people is not well developed and side effects are common. For these reasons psychiatric input to intervention is needed.

CATATONIA

Catatonia is a very specific and not uncommon problem in young people with autism. It presents with decreased mobility, sometimes to the extent that a person will stand in a fixed posture for long periods of time. Young people with catatonia are disinterested in their surroundings and interact even less than usual. Catatonia is more common when a young person is taking an antipsychotic medication, like risperidone, which may have been prescribed to assist with challenging behaviours not responding to behavioural interventions. Other drugs have also been implicated in the onset of catatonia, so a careful review of prescribed and non-prescribed drug intake is needed. Catatonia occurs in about 15 per cent of young people with autism (see Resources at the end of the chapter).

If a drug linked to catatonia is being taken it should be stopped, but in a staged way in consultation with the prescribing doctor. It may be that other medications will need to be started and again this should be done in a staged way with medical input.

EATING DISORDERS

Fussy eating has been discussed in Chapter 5 yet eating problems can emerge or continue in the teenage years. If your young person with autism starts to lose weight and continues to eat less than usual, it is important that you seek medical advice. A physical cause will need to be excluded along with underlying problems, such as depression (see above) or a fixed false belief (one type of psychotic thinking) and measures taken to ensure adequate nutrition.

ALCOHOL AND DRUGS

As your child gets older they may start drinking alcohol or taking recreational drugs. This often happens when young people are feeling confused, depressed or anxious. As described above, both prescribed and non-prescribed drugs can cause physical, emotional, behavioural and thought disorders so keep this in mind and ask about it if problems develop.

It is best to anticipate recreational alcohol or drug use as a potential problem and to explain to your young person with autism the hazards involved in a way they will understand. Even if the short-term experience is one they enjoy or one that helps them overcome social difficulties, there will be unwanted side effects. If they are able to understand this level of complexity, it is also best to explain to them that, even though they may have feelings and thoughts that make them want to escape, and experiences that make them feel worried or stressed, recreational drugs are not a good solution. Suggest instead that if they are feeling overwhelmed, sad, worried, isolated, unsupported or are having other troubling thoughts, visions or ideas, the best thing to do is to tell you or a professional that they trust, and to follow the advice they receive.

Much of what we've written about may never occur in your young person with autism. However, if it does, it is important to know that others have experienced the same problems and that strategies are available to deal with them.

LEAVING SCHOOL

The choices available for young people with autism will be different depending on the severity of their autism, the presence of any co-occurring conditions such as intellectual disability, or any co-morbid mental health issues, and the availability of post-school options. The majority of young people with autism continue to need some support in making the transition to employment or tertiary education and independent or supported living. Unfortunately, support services are limited even in the wealthiest countries. Services available for young people with autism and a significant intellectual disability, like John, are likely to be in the form of some kind of day program, possibly a supported employment program and supported accommodation, such as a group home in the community. Staff at specialist schools or units will be aware of the range of options available and the processes for accessing them and will discuss these with you in your young person's final years of school.

> Mike and Sue had hoped John would move into a supported employment program so he could work once he finished school, but although he was physically capable of work, his anxiety about any change and his limited communication meant that he needed high levels of support and supervision. John was assessed to determine the level of support funding he would receive. Mike and Sue were concerned to find that he was not allocated enough funding to attend the day program full time and was only able to go four days a week. Fortunately, they were able to negotiate a respite package as well which meant that he was allocated one weekend a month in a respite house, which gave them all a break.

Siew completed secondary school in the specialist autism unit and completed his leaving certificate. The staff in the unit introduced a transition program for Siew to his local technical college where he enrolled in a horticulture program with work experience with council mainenance crews in city parks and gardens. The staff, in collaboration with the teachers from the autism unit and Hong Yuan and Kenneth, set up a program for Siew to learn new skills and also to adapt the work crew processes to support Siew. For example, they set up the tool storage shed in an orderly way with shadow diagrams on the walls to show Siew where he needed to store the tools. The work crew were happy to make up a visual schedule for Siew showing the activities for the day.

For young people with autism in regular schools the possibilities are quite variable and usually under-resourced.

As Jane approached school-leaving age, staff at the school worked with Louise to find a place in an adult education setting where she could continue to develop her information technology skills. Jane was assessed by a specialist teacher to identify areas of strength and interest. The specialist teacher linked Jane into a supported adult education course and the local disability support service available in her area. Jane was also able to access disability income support because of Louise's financial situation as a sole carer. Considerations when choosing a pathway for Jane after school included her preference for vocational training in an occupation requiring repetitive and logical tasks — this played to her need for routine and minimised the risk of anxiety relating to change. Consideration was also given to a pathway that would avoid the need for interactions with customers. Although her diet had improved, consideration was still needed to ensure she had the ability to choose her own food to cater for her limited diet. The local community disability support service also linked Jane and Louise with a special interest social club for young adults with autism.

For young people like Todd there are often few services available to support transition to work or tertiary education.

Todd completed his schooling with high enough marks in his final exams to gain a place at university to study chemical engineering. He told Jessica and Joseph he didn't want to contact the disability support service at the university for help as he didn't think they would help students like him. Jessica and Joseph were delighted Todd had managed to get into the university course he wanted, but they were worried when they found out there was no specific support for students with autism at the university and wondered how he would cope without the supports that had been so important to his success at secondary school. Although Todd refused to register for formal support, he found a staff member in the maths department that he liked and trusted and met with him regularly, troubleshooting any problems he was having.

RESOURCES

Autism and the secondary school years

www.amaze.org.au/discover/about-autism-spectrum-disorder/
changing-to-high-school-the-high-school-years/

Questions for secondary schools

http://raisingchildren.net.au/articles/autism_spectrum_disorder_
choosing_school_teenagers.html

The hidden curriculum and making friends

www.education.com/reference/article/hidden-curriculum-school-
asperger/

www.autismtraining.com.au/orionfiles/upload/public/files/
informationsession_makingfriends.pdf

Advice about bullying, including cyber bullying

http://bullyingnoway.gov.au/

http://raisingchildren.net.au/articles/pip_cyberbullying.html/
context/1092

Sexuality and relationships

http://raisingchildren.net.au/articles/autism_spectrum_disorder_
sexuality_relationships_teenagers.html

Managing challenging behaviour

www.autism.org.uk/living-with-autism/understanding-behaviour/
challenging-behaviour/challenging-behaviour-in-children-with-an-
asd.aspx

A toolkit for managing challenging behaviours and the crises they can sometimes create

www.autismspeaks.org/family-services/tool-kits/challenging-
behaviors-tool-kit

The specific information about who to call is US-based, but the
general information and advice can be applied in other countries.

Medication for non-crisis management

http://onlinelibrary.wiley.com/doi/10.1002/14651858.CD005040.pub2/
abstract

http://raisingchildren.net.au/articles/atypical_antipsychotics_
th.html

Self-injuring behaviour

www.youthbeyondblue.com/understand-what's-going-on/self-harm-and-self-injury

www.autism.org.uk/living-with-autism/understanding-behaviour/challenging-behaviour/self-injurious-behaviour.aspx

Anxiety

www.adaa.org/understanding-anxiety/DSM-5-changes

www.headspace.org.au/what-works/research-information/anxiety

www.nice.org.uk/guidance/CG113/chapter/1-Guidance

Psychoses

www.headspace.org.au/what-works/research-information/psychosis

http://publications.nice.org.uk/psychosis-and-schizophrenia-in-children-and-young-people-cg155/recommendations

Catatonia

www.autismspeaks.org/blog/2014/01/03/does-our-teen-have-autism-related-catatonia

The hidden curriculum

Myles, B., Troutman, M., Schevlan, R. *The Hidden Curriculum: Practical solutions for understanding unstated rules in social situations*, Autism Asperger Publishing Co, Kansas, 2004.

CHAPTER 10

MAKING SENSE OF NEW INFORMATION

The way we access and share information has changed enormously in the past few decades, while the amount of information available has multiplied many times over. The 24-hour news cycle puts the very latest scientific breakthroughs in front of us, and the internet provides a seemingly endless trail to follow topics of interest. At the same time, scientific research is working harder to catch our attention. Modern scientists are under pressure to publish and promote their work to satisfy their funders and employers, with research into autism, in particular, booming. For a parent who is interested in keeping up with the field, the question is how to make sense of it all?

We hope in this chapter to provide some of the tools you'll need to assess the latest information about causes, diagnostic tools, treatments and outcomes.

SOURCES OF INFORMATION

Good starting points for further reading about findings relating to autism are systematic reviews, published guidelines and high quality websites, often run by research groups or government organisations.

Systematic reviews aim to survey all of the research undertaken about a particular topic and present an overall picture of what is known. The authors do a lot of work to ensure they find the right information and share it in an open manner. They develop search strategies to find all the relevant articles on a topic and ensure only those articles are included. They assess each study to decide if the study methods could have led to findings that are higher or lower (biased) than an ideal study would produce, and rate the overall quality of the evidence that is avilable to answer the question. The aim is to provide data to generate a meta-analysis, which is pooling sufficiently similar data to give an overall measure of what is known about a topic at the time of the review. So if you can find a systematic review that addresses a question you are interested in, you will have all the information you need in one article instead of having to read many different ones. Like any other scientific publication, systematic reviews should be read critically to ensure their methods include all the information that you consider relevant and also that no opportunity for bias has been introduced that would influence either the data that is included or the authors' interpretation of it (see Resources at the end of the chapter).

Guidelines are developed for a range of topics by countries and organisations to help policy makers, service planners and clinicians make the right decisions about best care. As a parent of a child or young person with autism, guidelines can be helpful for you too. To achieve a low risk of bias in the evidence presented in guidelines, the methods have to be available for you to review. This can make a guideline very long. However, increasingly, guidelines are being presented electronically and in a well-organised format so that you can move about them easily to find the bits that are relevant to you (for example, the guidelines about anxiety listed in the Resources for

Chapter 9). To date, we are not aware of one 'go to' guideline about autism. There are, however, increasing numbers of summaries about effective interventions (see Resources in Chapter 5), which organise multiple systematic reviews together so different interventions can be considered together. Also, there are some guidelines for ideal diagnostic pathways and procedures for autism (see Resources in Chapter 3), and a number of guidelines addressing problems associated with autism, like ADHD guidelines (see Resources in Chapter 8), that are useful.

Some excellent websites have also been developed to assist families. These websites present high-level evidence from systematic reviews and have guidelines embedded in them but they are presented in a more 'user friendly' way. Throughout the book we have referenced some of these resources and there is also a list at the end of this chapter.

Unfortunately, not all websites that exist are of a high quality. Some are designed to market an intervention, diagnostic approach or other service, although this purpose is not always immediately evident. Others are designed to present one perspective rather than a broad and balanced view. There are ways to assess websites to help you decide on their worth. These are fairly quick to apply once you get into the habit and can save you time in the long run. A few quick things you can ask yourself are: (1) is the information coming from qualified professionals and are the professionals' qualifications right for the topic?; (2) does anyone stand to benefit, financially or in other ways, if their view changes your opinion and/or actions?; (3) is there any evidence other than testimonials? and; (4) is there anything written on a website that I trust about this topic?

Another way to think about this is that marketing and advertising commonly target two emotions — hope and fear. If you feel flooded by hope or fear when reading material about causes, diagnostic tests and interventions for autism, it is most likely you have not been reading science or high-quality evidence.

Some reliable sources of information about autism and autism research are provided at the end of this chapter. Even within these reliable sources there will be different interpretations of the evidence and different recommendations found, further indicating how uncertain some things still are.

LOOKING AT EVIDENCE

When you read articles or scientific studies about autism, it can be helpful to keep in mind some broad concepts about how to gauge the worth of the information before you. Many things proven in scientific articles are later 'disproven' or discredited. This is because science is always evolving as our existing knowledge is built upon or challenged. There are also reasons why findings that are not yet proven are presented as though they are. Some scientists are under pressure to publish in order to improve their reputation and even salary or position, so they will publish early results. Early results are much more likely to show an association or positive effect for an intervention. They wouldn't get published if they didn't. This is known as publication bias. Early studies are likely to use 'test the water' methods that are less scientifically sound for the question at hand, for example open-label drug trials versus a randomised drug trial, in which the participants and the professionals who assess outcomes do not know whether they are receiving the interventions. It is also known that less rigorous methods are likely to yield positive results, rather than 'no effect' or 'no association' results, and when there is a positive effect or association it is likely to be of a higher magnitude. Also, many things that are presented at conferences are 'preliminary' analyses. This sort of data is the same as the 'early publication' data and much more likely to show strong associations or positive intervention effects when later analyses with larger samples show none.

Since the early 1990s, there has been added clarity in the way we think about the types of evidence we need to make decisions about health care. The movement started with the concept of 'clinical epidemiology'. Epidemiology studies the prevalence, cause and control of disease in large populations. Clinical epidemiology describes the types of information we need to make clinical care decisions — information about cause, diagnosis, prognosis and intervention, and the ideal types of scientific studies to provide that information. The application of clinical epidemiology to medicine became known as evidence-based medicine. The idea is that all the available evidence to answer an important clinical question should be assessed to ensure it is providing an estimate that is close to the 'truth' before it is applied to health care. Whether existing evidence is a good estimate of the 'truth' depends on how free of bias it is and whether chance alone could have explained the findings. To assess these things you need to read articles with an analytical or critical perspective.

You might be interested in reading a publication of an individual study if a systematic review or guideline is not yet available. Table 4 lists the different types of questions that you might be asking, the optimal study design for answering that question, and key features and findings to look out for.

Table 4: Study designs and the questions they can answer

Questions	Optimal study design	Where to find more information including how to assess the study you read
Is an intervention effective compared to no intervention or an alternative intervention?	Controlled trials, ideally randomised	» www.cebm.net/critical-appraisal/ and click on Therapy/RCT under Critical Appraisal Worksheets » www.healthknowledge.org.uk/public-health-textbook/research-methods/1a-epidemiology/cs-as-is/intervention-studies-rct » www.asatonline.org/research-treatment/evaluating-research/

What is the cause?	Prospective cohort studies	» www.asatonline.org/research-treatment/making-sense-of-autism-treatments-weighing-the-evidence/what-caused-that/
		» www.healthknowledge.org.uk/public-health-textbook/research-methods/1a-epidemiology/cs-as-is/case-control-studies
		» www.healthknowledge.org.uk/public-health-textbook/research-methods/1a-epidemiology/association-causation
Will this test provide useful information?	Diagnostic test accuracy studies	» www.cebm.net/critical-appraisal/ and click on Diagnosis under Critical Appraisal Worksheets
		» http://guides.mclibrary.duke.edu/content.p?pid=431451&sid=3530520
What is the outcome (prognosis)?	Prospective follow-up studies	» www.cebm.net/critical-appraisal/ and click on Prognosis under Critical Appraisal Worksheets
		» http://guides.mclibrary.duke.edu/content.php?pid=431451&sid=3530525
		» www.healthknowledge.org.uk/public-health-textbook/research-methods/1a-epidemiology/sudies-disease-prognosis

How common is this problem?	Population-based with clinical validation of those identified	» www.healthknowledge.org.uk/public-health-textbook/research-methods/1a-epidemiology/cs-as-is/cross-sectional-studies » http://sfari.org/news-and-opinion/viewpoint/2012/population-based-studies-key-for-assessing-autism-prevalence

THE DIFFICULTY OF DECISION-MAKING

Making decisions when much is still uncertain is difficult. Even when the positive effects of an intervention are well known or a diagnostic test is known to be very accurate, there are still many other factors that might influence your choice of an intervention or whether or not to have a test, like a genetic test or MRI. Our advice is to think carefully about what you would like to achieve.

INTERVENTION

With an intervention, know what your goals are for yourself or your child. Think about the goals in more detail. Are they realistic? How would you know if they are met? What timeframe would be reasonable to expect them to be achieved? Talk to others about these goals. If the goals are educational, then your child's teacher is a good person to ask. Friends and family might also bring interesting perspectives.

Now think about the intervention. There will always be risks, so what are they? If it is a medication, your doctor will know what the risks are and how likely they are to occur. For other interventions there may not be well-documented risk, but the intervention might prevent the family engaging in time together, might cost money that increases family stress, or might require that you spend time away from work. Think about these things too. If your child is young you should factor in that some risks are greater and longer lasting for young children, where factors of growth and learning increase vulnerability.

If you decide to go ahead with an intervention, make a record of what your goals are and keep a record of your child's progress. Decide on how and how often you will record information about whether a goal has been met or if there is progress towards it. For example, you might record once a week how often an unwanted behaviour has happened that day. Get someone else who cares for your child or works with them to record progress too, ideally in a different setting, like school or day care. Everyone is too busy to remember what has happened over a period of a few weeks, and in autism you are likely to be looking for change over a longer period than that.

Remember to refer back to your goals at intervals and to use that as an opportunity to make decisions about continuing or stopping an intervention.

TESTS

For a test (such as a genetic test or MRI) to be useful, you need to understand what the test is able to achieve and what it is not able to achieve and also whether having the information that the test provides will change what happens next. Tests that do not have the potential to change your understanding of things or what happens next are not useful. Like interventions, all tests have associated possible harms, some more than others. As you are presented with possible tests for your child or young person with autism, it is very reasonable for you to ask about and think through what the test results could be and how or whether they would change the future for you and your family. You should also think about whether you value the sort of information that can be provided and how you might act if you have that information. This can be different for different people. Some prefer the 'what you don't know can't hurt you' and 'ignorance is bliss' approach. Others can't function unless all the details are available, and prefer knowing to not knowing regardless of whether the answer is good news or not. Most people are a bit of both and react differently for different types of information. You and your partner might have different approaches to this, so it is good to discuss each other's views and factor that into your decision-making.

CAUSES

When you are trying to decide if something causes autism you are probably really deciding if you should consider whether your child has a test or starts an intervention. In the science or evidence cycle, a theory about a cause needs to follow many steps to become a proven cause (see Chapter 1). Once something has been established as a cause then further steps are needed to assess whether a diagnostic test correctly identifies that cause and whether an intervention targeting that cause is effective. That cycle can take a long time and many parents don't feel they have the time to wait to make a decision. If you feel you are in that position, you need to closely examine all the risks of the test or intervention, both in the short and long term. You may be a risk-taker or risk-averse. Recognise this quality in yourself and remember that you are acting on behalf of another person as you make this decision, because as their parent you have discretion over most aspects of your child's care. The bottom line is that, in the absence of evidence, you should cause no harm and avoid incurring costs (financial or others, like losing family time) that you can't afford (see Resources at the end of the chapter).

It is hard to know what decision you make today you might regret tomorrow, but it is true that more is not always better and action is as often regretted as inaction.

RESOURCES

Genetic discoveries, research in the news and a summary of 'what we know'

http://sfari.org/

Systematic reviews about autism and related problems

www.thecochranelibrary.com/details/browseReviews/579405/
Autistic-spectrum-disorder.html

Guidelines about autism

www.nice.org.uk/Guidance/Conditions-and-diseases/Mental-health-
and-behavioural-conditions/Autism

www.health.govt.nz/publication/new-zealand-autism-spectrum-
disorder-guideline

Evidence summaries about cause, diagnosis and interventions for autism

www.researchautism.net/

Evidence summaries about interventions, as well as general information about autism and the stages of childhood

http://raisingchildren.net.au/children_with_autism/children_with_
autism_spectrum_disorder.html

www.researchautism.net/

Evidence-based practices

http://autismpdc.fpg.unc.edu/content/ebp-update

http://effectivehealthcare.ahrq.gov/index.cfm/search-for-guides-
reviews-and-reports/?productid=1945&pageaction=displayproduct

Provides useful reviews when there is media coverage about autism research

www.nhs.uk/News/Pages/NewsIndex.aspx

Information about using evidence for decision-making and choosing interventions as well as other specific information via the homepage

www.positivepartnerships.com.au/en/fact-sheet/using-evidence-
guide-decision-making

Further reading about assessing information and studies about autism

www.autismspectrumexplained.com/how-to-assess-claims.html

PARTING WORDS

We hope that writing about the things we've learnt while working with children, young people and their families has gathered together information in a way that will help you. We've met so many amazing children and young people with autism, and so many amazing parents. We know that living with children and young people with autism brings additional challenges for parents, siblings and others who are close to them. We know that you'll make decisions you regret, that you'll worry about the future and that you'll realise there are things that you'd like to influence but you can't.

Just as there is no one type of person with autism, there is no one type of family or one type of journey. Nor is there one right way of providing best care and support and opportunities for success. If you are taking positive steps to try to understand your child and their needs, if you are there for them and doing everything you can to keep them safe and well, then you're doing a great job!

We hope you meet many excellent professionals who can assist you during the different ages and stages of your child and young person's life and that over time you have much to celebrate. Don't expect too much of yourself and don't be afraid to ask for help as you work with those around you to be the sort of parent you want to be.

ENDNOTES

CHAPTER 1: WHAT IS AUTISM?

1. American Psychiatric Association. *Diagnostic and Statistical Manual of Mental Disorders* (4th edn), Washington, DC: American Psychiatric Association, 1994. www.dsm.psychiatryonline.org (pervasive developmental disorders): accessed 1 June 2013.

2. World Health Organization. International Statistical Classification of Diseases and Related Health Problems (10th revision), Geneva, 2010. http://apps.who.int/classifications/icd10/browse/2010/en#/F84.0.

3. American Psychiatric Association. *Diagnostic and Statistical Manual of Mental Disorders* (5th edn), Arlington, VA: American Psychiatric Publishing, 2013. www.dsm.psychiatryonline.org (autism spectrum disorder): accessed 1 June 2013.

4. www.ncbi.nlm.nih.gov/pmc/articles/PMC3763210/pdf/aur0005-0160.pdf: accessed 14 November 2014.

5. American Psychiatric Association. *Diagnostic and Statistical Manual of Mental Disorders* (4th edn), 1994.

6. American Psychiatric Association. *Diagnostic and Statistical Manual of Mental Disorders* (5th edn), 2013.

CHAPTER 3: ASSESSMENT AND DIAGNOSIS

1. American Psychiatric Association. *Diagnostic and Statistical Manual of Mental Disorders* (5th edn), Arlington, VA: American Psychiatric Publishing, 2013. www.dsm.psychiatryonline.org (autism spectrum disorder): accessed 1 June 2013.

2. American Psychiatric Association. *Diagnostic and Statistical Manual of Mental Disorders* (5th edn), 2013.

3. World Health Organization. International Statistical Classification of Diseases and Related Health Problems (10th revision), Geneva, 2010. http://apps.who.int/classifications/icd10/browse/2010/en#/F84.0.

4. American Psychiatric Association. *Diagnostic and Statistical Manual of Mental Disorders* (5th edn), 2013.

5. American Psychiatric Association. *Diagnostic and Statistical Manual of Mental Disorders* (5th edn), 2013.

6. American Psychiatric Association. *Diagnostic and Statistical Manual of Mental Disorders* (5th edn), 2013.

CHAPTER 5: THE TODDLER AND PRESCHOOL YEARS

1. Posted on a discussion forum on the *Positive Partnerships* website, 2008.

2. Prior, M. and Roberts, J. *Early Intervention for Children with Autism Spectrum Disorders: Guidelines for best practice*. Australian Government Department of Health and Ageing, Australia, 2006.

CHAPTER 7: THE PRIMARY SCHOOL YEARS

1. Jackson, Luke. *Freaks, Geeks and Asperger Syndrome. A user guide to adolescence*, Jessica Kingsley Publishers, London, 2002, p 134.

2. Lilley, Rozanna. 'Crying in the park: Autism stigma, school entry and maternal subjectivity', *Studies in the Maternal*, 5(2), 2013. www.mamsie.bbk.ac.uk/documents/Lilley_SiM_5(2)2013.pdf2: accessed 24 October 2014.

3. Personal communication from a parent of a six-year-old in a regular classroom.

CHAPTER 8: PROBLEMS IN THE PRIMARY SCHOOL YEARS

1. American Psychiatric Association. *Diagnostic and Statistical Manual of Mental Disorders* (5th edn), Arlington, VA: American Psychiatric Publishing, 2013. www.dsm.psychiatryonline.org (attention-deficit/hyperactivity disorder): accessed 1 June 2013.

2. American Psychiatric Association. *Diagnostic and Statistical Manual of Mental Disorders* (5th edn), 2013.

CHAPTER 9: THE SECONDARY SCHOOL YEARS

1. Sainsbury, Clare. *Martian in the Playground: Understanding the schoolchild with Asperger's Syndrome* (2nd edn), SAGE Publications Ltd, London, 2009.

GLOSSARY

Acceptance and commitment therapy (ACT)
> A relatively new approach promoting the principles of mindfulness and identifying and connecting with one's personal values in order to cope with difficult situations.

Applied behavioural analysis (ABA)
> An intervention based on the idea that you can change behaviour by analysing and changing the antecedent (trigger) or the consequence, and that by reinforcing wanted behaviour you increase the likelihood of it reoccurring. ABA is the basis of many interventions for children with autism that involve teaching appropriate behaviour by breaking down complex tasks into smaller, more achievable steps and rewarding a correct response. A skill might be taught in a series of small steps called discrete trials (stimulus–response–reinforcement), which are repeated many times.

Asperger's syndrome/Asperger's disorder
> The diagnostic term used in some classification systems (but no longer included in *DSM-5*) for individuals with average or above average intelligence and language development who have low function in social communication, inflexibility and very restricted activities and interests sufficient to cause problems.

Attention deficit hyperactivity disorder (ADHD)
> A diagnostic term characterising problems with concentrating and attending to tasks accompanied by needing to be up and 'on the go', all of which are more than expected for a person's age.

Atypical autism
> A diagnostic term used in the International Classification of Diseases system (ICD) to describe individuals with features common in other types of autism, but in whom some of the features are different, like a later age of onset.

Auditory Integration Training (AIT)

A therapy in which a child wears headphones and listens to music that has been filtered (attenuating sounds at selected frequencies) and/or modulated (random alternating of high and low sounds). Aimed at increasing or decreasing sound sensitivities to certain frequencies.

Augmentative and alternative communication (AAC)

A term used to describe all communication that is not speech, which can be used to enhance or replace speech when there are problems with that form of communication. Examples of AAC include gestures, eye pointing, vocalisations and pointing to symbols, including written words.

Autism

The shortened umbrella term used for many other diagnoses like autism spectrum disorder, Asperger's syndrome, atypical autism, autistic disorder and childhood autism. It is used to define a combination of problems associated with social communication and behaviours that include some but not necessarily all of the following: resistance to change; highly restricted interests and activities; repetitive behaviours; and over-or under-sensitivity to sensory stimuli, like sounds.

Autism Diagnostic Interview and its versions (ADI, ADI-R, ADI-2)

An interview that asks specific questions about current and past behaviours in a certain way to assist with the diagnosis of autism. Currently it is widely used in clinical care and research.

Autism Diagnostic Observation Schedule and its versions (ADOS, ADOS-G, ADOS-Module T (Toddler), Prelinguistic (PL-ADOS, ADOS-2)

An assessment that uses specific toys, pictures and other prompts to elicit behaviours which the examiner observes and decides if they are within the normal range for ability and age. The ADOS focuses on behaviours that are directly linked to the diagnosis of autism. There have been many versions and the latest incorporates modules for all ages and abilities.

Autism spectrum disorders (ASD)

A term used since the 1980s to bring together under one term all people who have problems in social communication and behaviours described above for autism. Since 2013, this is the official diagnostic term for the *DSM-5* classification system.

Checklist for Autism in Toddlers and its versions (CHAT, M–CHAT, M-CHAT-R)

A tool designed to be applied to whole populations of children to identify those with problems that could indicate that they have autism before parents or clinicians have raised concerns. Some clinicians use the CHAT or its versions if a parent raises concerns about their child's development to be sure they have asked questions about autism.

Childhood Autism Rating Scale and its versions (CARS, CARS-2)

A combination of specific questions and observations of certain behaviours to assist with the diagnosis of autism. The CARS was one of the first interview and observation tools developed for autism and is widely used for clinical assessment and research.

Clinical trial

A research study in which a treatment is being investigated to assess whether it is effective.

Cognition and cognitive

Cognition is the ability to think and includes all the mental activities and processes required for thinking, such as remembering things, concentrating and interpreting sensory input. It enables a person to problem-solve and empathise.

Cognitive behaviour therapy

An established psychological therapy that provides practical strategies to challenge or change unhelpful or unhealthy thoughts or behaviours to enable an individual to cope in a situation in which problems have occurred.

Developmental assessment

An assessment that uses specific toys, pictures and other prompts so all areas of development can be observed and assessed. Key areas of a developmental assessment include physical ability, manipulation of small objects, communication, self-care and the ability to reason and solve puzzles.

Developmental, Dimensional and Diagnostic Interview (3di)

An interview that asks specific questions in a certain way to assist with the diagnosis of autism and also assesses problems that are commonly associated with autism.

Developmental disorder

A lack in the appearance of skills in one or more areas of development that is outside the usual range expected for a child's age.

Diagnostic and Statistical Manual of Mental Disorders (DSM)

A classification system for conditions that are diagnosed based on mood, thoughts or behaviours.

Diagnostic Interview for Social and Communication Disorders (DISCO)

An interview that asks specific questions in a certain way to assist with the diagnosis of autism and also gathers information about skills and other key aspects of behaviour and development.

Developmental, Individual Difference, Relationship-based (DIR®) model and DIRFloortime®

A model for assessment that directly links to an intervention approach. It is based on a child's developmental challenges and strengths, and builds on relationships. DIRFloortime® is a particular technique based on developing abilities that are necessary for social communication by engaging the child and following the child's lead.

Discrete Trial Training (DTT)

A series of stimulus–response–reinforcement steps and a pause. Training involves repeating this sequence.

DNA

DNA is the abbreviation for deoxyribonucleic acid. It is the fundamental structural element of all our cells. It gives the instructions that change the development and growth of different cell types and direct how they work.

Dyspraxia

There is no internationally agreed definition for dyspraxia. Some people use it interchangeably with developmental motor coordination disorder, which is now included in *DSM-5* and indicates difficulties with coordinated movement that are not due to other diagnosable physical, sensory or intelligence problems.

Early Start Denver Model (ESDM)

An early intervention program designed for use in a child's usual environments, including groups. It is based on developmental, behavioural and relationship-based strategies that are described in a manual but tailored for each child's abilities and challenges.

Echolalia

The repetition of speech either just heard or heard in the past. It is described as imitation in young children and is part of learning to talk, however if it persists and occurs frequently after the child is three years of age, it is described as echolalia.

Education or learning plan

A plan that is developed to cater to a student's unique strengths and needs to optimise their learning and participation in their educational setting. It is developed by bringing together information from everyone who knows the student well, including the student whenever possible.

Electroencephalogram (EEG)

A test that measures the electrical activity of the brain and assesses whether there is electrical activity that is known to trigger seizures (also known as convulsions).

Epidemiology

The study of health and disease patterns in populations. Epidemiological studies provide information about the incidence and prevalence of problems, and the risk factors for health conditions. This information is used to plan preventive approaches and to form service planning and public health policy.

Epigenetics

The study of DNA in the regions surrounding the genes, known as epigenetic regions. Genes can be made to function differently by the DNA located near them, even though the gene itself is not different to the gene in other people. DNA in epigentic regions can turn genes on and off permanently or for short periods.

Epilepsy

The label given to recurring seizures that are not triggered by fever or fainting or other known physiological problems, like low blood sugar.

Evidence/evidence-based

Evidence is information from well-conducted studies that have used the right design to answer a question or test a hypothesis. Evidence-based refers to practice, service development or policy that uses relevant evidence to make decision, about what is best.

Expressive communication

The way we convey what we mean to other people either by using spoken words, gestures, movements, images or text.

Fine motor skills

The skills we use to manipulate small objects, which allows us to write and use tools. Fine motor skills require normal sensation, muscle strength and coordination.

Gilliam Autism Rating Scale and its versions (GARS, GARS-2, GARS-3)

An interview that asks specific questions about autism-related behaviours in a certain way to assist identifying the probability of a child having autism and also to indicate the severity.

Gluten and casein free (GFCF) diet

A diet that is free from gluten (a key component of wheat) and casein (a key component of milk and other dairy foods).

Gross motor skills

The skills we use for walking, running, hopping and climbing stairs. Normal sensation and muscle strength are needed as well as messages from the brain to tell you where your limbs are.

High-functioning autism

A term often used to describe people with autism who have normal or above average intelligence. There is ongoing controversy about whether high functioning autism can be distinguished from Asperger's syndrome.

Hyper-reactivity (also described as hyper-sensitive)

An over-reaction to sensory input in any one or more of the senses (hearing, sight, taste, smell, touch, balance or sense of body in space). Can include becoming upset at some sounds, some visual stimuli, and also avoidance of some activities involving touch.

Hyporeactivity (also described as hyposensitive)

An under-reaction to sensory input in any one or more of the senses (hearing, sight, taste, smell, touch, balance or sense of body in space). A less common example of hyporeactivity is indifference to pain.

Intellectual disability

A term used to describe problems with thinking that impact function. Other terms used include 'intellectual impairment', 'learning disability' and in the past 'mental retardation'.

Intelligence quotient (IQ)

A quotient or score calculated after completing an intelligence test using accepted tools that compare the score achieved with what is expected for age. Domains include practical reasoning and verbal ability.

Intensive Behavioural Intervention (IBI)/Early Intensive Behavioural Intervention (EIBI)

A term used for interventions that are based on ABA which are delivered either one-on-one or in groups. The intensiveness of the intervention refers to the number of hours that the program is delivered, with many programs scheduling twenty or more hours per week of intervention. If delivered in the preschool years this is often called Early Intensive Behavioural Intervention (EIBI).

International Classification of Diseases (ICD-10)

A classification system for conditions that are diagnosed based on physical and biological problems as well as problems with mood, thoughts or behaviours. As such, it includes conditions that appear in the DSM classification system as well as problems with known biological causes that do not affect the brain or mind.

Intervention

A broad term used for all activities designed to improve a condition or problem. Interventions can include drugs, physical therapies, complementary and alternative therapies, educational, developmental and behavioural approaches or environmental changes. Other terms used that are all interventions include treatment, therapy and program.

Joint attention *see* Shared attention

Low-functioning autism

A term often used to describe people with autism who have low functional intelligence.

Magnetic resonance imaging (MRI)/Functional magnetic resonance imaging (fMRI)

A test that uses magnetic fields and radio waves to visualise internal organs and structures to find, or rule out, problems. Functional MRI assesses how organs, like the brain, are working by visualising differences in blood flow.

Mainstream

A term used to describe schools that are open to all children without specific entry criteria. These are also known as regular schools.

Melatonin

A hormone that is secreted by the pineal gland, with increased secretion when it is dark. Melatonin is best known for its role in the sleep–wake cycle with increased melatonin linked to sleep. Melatonin interacts with other hormones and some of its roles are still being discovered.

Meta-analysis

A method of statistical analysis that brings together data from different studies to provide an overall estimate, taking into account differences in sample size and effect size of the included studies. Like other statistical techniques there are instances in which meta-analysis should not be used

Mindfulness

An approach adapted from Buddhist mindfulness meditation that focuses on the present time and accepting rather than judging the way things are. Mindfulness is now being incorporated into psychological therapies like ACT.

Motor planning

The ability to plan motor activities, like picking up a cup, once you have the idea of what you want to do. For planned motor activities to be executed other thought processes, like sensory awareness and memory, are needed and muscle strength and coordination is also required.

Multidisciplinary

An approach based on bringing together professionals from different disciplines to find the best solutions to complex problems. In autism, multidisciplinary teams are needed for assessment and diagnosis as well as intervention.

Neurodevelopmental

Refers to brain development and the behaviours and abilities we know are needed for proper development of the brain. Neurodevelopmental disorders are impairments of the development of the brain and central nervous system.

Neurological

Refers to all systems involving the nerve cells in our body. This includes the brain, the nerves that travel to our limbs and the nerves that control how our organs work.

Neuropsychology

A branch or subspecialty of psychology that focuses on brain functions like memory, problem-solving, attention and concentration, and planning. Neuropsychologists provide assessment of brain functions and approaches to manage behaviours related to brain functioning.

Neurotypical

A term coined by people with autism describing people who do not have autism. The use of the term implies that autism can be considered to be a difference rather than a disability and draws attention to the fact that 'autism' and 'typical' (or 'normal') are relative constructs rather than absolute ones.

Obsessive compulsive disorder (OCD)

A diagnosis used when a person becomes preoccupied with a thought in a way that impedes their ability to function normally. The preoccupying thought will drive actions which lead to the problems the person experiences. For example, a fear of infections might lead to a person never going out or to repetitive hand washing (a compulsion).

Peer review

A process in which scientific study (research), reports or plans are critically reviewed by colleagues with expertise in the same topic or in the methods used for research design or statistical analysis that will or have been used. In this process a report or planned study will receive feedback and either be published or funded, or not.

Pervasive developmental disorder–not otherwise specified (PDD–NOS)

A diagnostic label in *DSM-IV* for people who had the same sort of behaviours as people diagnosed with Autistic Disorder, but fewer of them. The equivalent term in ICD-10 is Pervasive developmental disorder, unspecified. Neither diagnoses specified the number of behavioural criteria needed.

Pica

The act of persistently eating items that are not considered food.

Picture Exchange Communication System (PECS)

An augmentative and alternative communication (AAC) system often used to teach communication skills to children with autism. The child is taught to initiate a request by giving an adult a picture of what they want. For example, they learn to give a picture of a cup to request a drink. Once the child has learnt to give a picture (symbol) for an item they learn different symbols for what they want.

Pivotal Response Training (PRT)

Derived from ABA and developmental approaches, PRT is a play-based intervention that targets what its developers consider the pivotal aspects of child development: motivation, response to multiple cues, self-management and the initiation of social interactions. PRT strategies are incorporated into intervention programs, including the Early Start Denver Model (ESDM).

Placebo/Placebo effect

A placebo is an imitation or substitute for an intervention that is being tested, like a sugar pill compared to a medication, or unstructured play compared to a behavioural intervention. Placebos are used so a direct comparison can be made between people who receive the intervention that is being tested and those who are not.

Pragmatics

A term used to describe the function or purpose of communication. Primary functions of communication are request/demand, reject, protest, sharing information and greeting. The term pragmatics can also refer to the multiple and subtle rules that govern human conversations, and the ability of speakers to adjust their language depending on context and their conversation partner.

Prevalence

The proportion of the population with a condition. It includes all people with the problem in a given location over a specified period of time. Birth prevalence is the proportion of people who were born in a given year who have a condition. Incidence differs from prevalence by including only people who are newly identified.

Proprioception

The sense of where our body parts are in relation to each other and other items in our environment, like the floor and desktop. Proprioception is important for gross and fine motor skills and motor planning.

Randomised controlled trial

A clinical trial or study that randomly allocates people to receive one intervention versus another (such as another active intervention or a placebo). This method is used to achieve an even spread of features that could influence whether a person responds to the intervention or not across the two or more groups. In doing this it reduces potential bias in the study.

Receptive communication

The way we are able to understand the communication of others. This includes spoken words, gestures, movements, images or text.

Relationship Development Intervention (RDI)®

A parent-led autism therapy aimed at developing social relationships, starting with the immediate family.

Rett syndrome

> A genetic disorder that affects mainly girls. Behaviours in the preschool years are similar to those seen in autism, but the course is one of loss of skills and decline in physical wellbeing.

Savant skills (also known as splinter skills)

> Skills that are developed beyond what would be expected for age and are out of keeping with ability in other areas.

Selective serotonin reuptake inhibitors (SSRIs)

> A group of drugs that inhibit the reuptake of serotonin at nerve junctions. The listed indications for their use in children and young people differs between countries. They have a role in the management of OCD and depression when used as an adjunct to effective behavioural interventions when a problem is severe or not responding to usual therapy.

Self-stimulatory behaviour/Stimming

> Repetitive body movements that can also involve the movement of objects to stimulate the senses. Also called sterotypies, the action is commonly referred to as 'stimming'. The function of self-stimulating behaviours is varied and may differ from person to person and even in one person for different behaviours and the same behaviour in different situations. Self-stimulatory behaviours may be used to block out distressing input, as a self-calming behaviour, or because they provide a pleasurable sensory experience.

Sensory integration therapy

> A type of intervention that uses sensory inputs to improve the processing of one or more sensations in the brain so that children learn to use all their senses together. Designed as a first step towards improved learning and behaviours. Stimulation of vestibular (balance), tactile (touch), and/or proprioceptive (sense of where the body is in space) senses could include swinging in a hammock, balancing on beams, and brushing or stroking.

Sensory processing disorder

> A term used by some professionals to describe individuals with over- or underactive sensory perception or sensory distortions, in one or more of the senses. Although sensory problems are one criteria for a diagnosis of autism spectrum disorder in *DSM-5*, sensory processing disorder is not yet a formal diagnosis and does not appear in *DSM-5*.

Shared attention (also known as joint attention)

A key part of communication and underpins the development of language. It is the ability to share attention with another person either through eye contact, gesture, sound or words. Children learn to initiate joint attention, show another person something, and respond to joint attention when shown something by another person at an early age. Turn-taking also requires shared attention. Shared attention has a communicative purpose that is more than indicating a need.

Stereotypy

Repetitive movements without a clear purpose. Stereotypies can be self-stimulating.

Stimming *see* Self-stimulatory behaviour

Social stories

A short story that uses an explicit format and guidelines to describe a person, skill, event, concept or social situation. Used to support social interactions for children and young people with autism spectrum disorder by explaining the what, when, who and why of social situations and acceptable ways to behave.

Systematic review

Studies that aim to survey all of the research undertaken that could assist in answering a specific question and by doing this to present an overall picture of what is known. They differ from non-systematic reviews in that the authors do a lot of work to ensure they find all the relevant information on a topic and share it in an open manner. In a systematic review risk of bias is assessed for each included study. The aim is to provide data so the reader can see at a glance what evidence is currently available. In some systematic reviews a meta-analysis will be possible.

TEACCH®

An intensive, individually adapted intervention developed in the 1960s that creates a structured learning environment, including clear schedules of activities.

Theory of mind

The understanding that other people have thoughts and feelings that are different from one's own. The ability to infer from behaviours what others are thinking or feeling.

Tic

An intermittent, sudden and involuntary movement, such as grimacing or blinking, or vocalisation, like throat clearing.

Tourette's disorder

A tic disorder. A person diagnosed with Tourette's disorder (also known as Tourette's syndrome) will have multiple tics, both motor and vocal, that started before they were aged eighteen and have persisted for more than twelve months. Other causes of intermittent, sudden and involuntary movements, like drug side effects and seizures, must not be the cause of the movements.

Tuberous sclerosis

A genetic disorder in which benign tumours grow in the brain and other parts of the body. People with tuberous sclerosis can have seizures that are difficult to control in the first year of life. A higher proportion than expected have autism.

Vestibular

Refers to the system that is in the ear, with nerves running to the brain, which processes sensory information that is important for the control of balance.

Visual supports

Any item, such as an actual object, photo, picture or cartoon, that can be looked at rather than listened to. Visual supports can be used for expressive and receptive communication, as a point of reference to make things more predictable (for example, a visual schedule of the day's activities), to plan for change and to indicate boundaries or limits. Visual supports are used to help people with autism communicate, develop language and process information.

Visuospatial skills

The ability to visually perceive objects and the spatial relationships among objects. As with other skills people vary in their visuospatial abilities.

ACKNOWLEDGEMENTS

We'd like to dedicate this book to the parents, children and young people who we have known over the years and who have shared their stories with us. It has been a privilege to be a small part of your lives. We have learnt so much from you all — not only about autism, but about courage and not giving up and about what it means to be human.

We'd like to thank Exisle Publishing for suggesting the book to us and being flexible about submission dates. Thanks also to Richard Pullin for showing us how to turn science, education and health into something readable and to Lawrie Bartak, Catherine Marraffa and Vivian Bayl for their usual wise suggestions. We'd also like to thank Monica Berton for her editorial improvements, which included a crucial parent perspective.

And thanks also to all the people who have taught us about research, child development and autism, and to those who work with us today — all generous and clever people dreaming large about what the future could be like.

Thanks most of all to our families.

From Katrina: To my parents and brother for my fabulous early years and ongoing relationships. To Richard for so much support in so many things and to my wonderful children for making life so much more.

From Jacqui: To my family and especially to David and to Tim, for all your unwavering love, support and encouragement and for coping with all the times I wasn't there for you.

INDEX

drugs, recreational 189
DSM-5
    ADHD criteria 152–3
    autism/ADHD classification 151
    criteria and rules 40–2
    latest diagnosis criteria 53–5
    severity levels 41–2
DSM-IV, broadened diagnosis 11
dyspraxia 214

E

Early Intensive Behavioural Intervention
    (EIBI) 216
early intervention professional 31
early interventions
    different types 86–7
    evidence for 92–6
    guidelines for good practices 98
    key features 94–5
    website resources 97–8
Early Start Denver Model (ESDM) 214
eating
    changing fussy habits 122–3
    fussy/picky 119–23, 128
    non-food substances 125
eating disorders 189
echolalia 43, 214
education plan 214
electroencephalogram (EEG) 156, 214
emotional responses, recognising 174
emotions
    limited understanding 171
    recognition/regulation 140, 149
engagement, essential for development
    75–7
epidemiology 214
epigenetic regions
    change gene functions 7
    role in health problems 8–9
epigenetics 215
epilepsy 30, 154–6, 215
evidence-based practices 204, 215
executive function 48–9
expressive communication 215

F

families
    bilingual 77–8
    impact of diagnosis 64–5
    intervention involvement 95
fight or flight response 110
fine motor skills 215
food allergies 63, 121

website resources 128
food intolerances 121, 128
food separation 122–3
foods, tastes and textures 122
*Freaks, Geeks and Asperger Syndrome. A
    user guide to adolescence* (book) 129
friends, making 193
functional magnetic resonance imaging
    (fMRI) 217
fussy eating 119–23, 128

G

gagging, during meals 121
generalisation, difficulty with 85
genes
    as a cause 6, 50
    deletion/duplication 7
    research and findings 13
genetic changes, types of 7
genetic discoveries 204
genetic testing 50
Gilliam Autism Rating Scale (GARS) 215
gluten-free diet 123–4, 128, 215
grandmother, non-acceptance of diagnosis
    26
gross motor skills 215
guidelines
    developing 196–7
    website resources 204
guilt, parents' feelings of 63, 65–6

H

head banging 180
hearing test 49–50
hidden curriculum
    explained 171
    resources 194
    website resources 193
high-functioning autism 216
hitting 113–15
homework assignments 176
hyper-reactivity 216
hyporeactivity 216

I

imitation
    essential for development 75–7
    in speech 43
information sources
    looking at evidence 198–9
    range of 196–7
    study design and questions *199–201*